Handbook of
Endocrine Investigations in Children

Handbooks of Investigation in Children

This is a series of unique guides to the appropriate tests to be carried out in children with suspected disorders. Instructions for the performance and evaluation of tests are clearly explained. Each title is based on the authors' personal experience in the respective field and is devoted to the investigation of children only.

Careful reference to these titles in clinical practice will help both to eliminate inadequate testing and to ensure that the practitioner will obtain the maximum information from the investigations carried out. To amplify the explicit text, case histories helpfully illustrate how the authors have used and interpreted investigations. These pocket-sized books are essential tools for all those involved in the diagnosis and management of childhood disorders.

Other titles

Handbook of Haematological Investigations in Children
    R. F. Stevens
Handbook of Neurological Investigations in Children
    C. M. Taylor and S. Chapman
Handbook of Renal Investigations in Children
    J. B. P. Stephenson and M. D. King

Handbook of Endocrine Investigations in Children

I. A. HUGHES MD, FRCP, FRCP(C)
Reader in Paediatric Endocrinology
University of Wales College of Medicine, Cardiff and
Professor-Elect of Paediatrics, University of Cambridge

with a foreword by
Professor R. HALL

WRIGHT
London Boston Singapore Sydney Toronto Wellington

Wright
is an imprint of Butterworth Scientific

 PART OF REED INTERNATIONAL P.L.C.

First published 1986
Reprinted with revisions 1989

© **Butterworth & Co. (Publishers) Ltd, 1986**

British Library Cataloguing in Publication Data

Hughes, I. A.
    Handbook of endocrine investigations in children.
    1. Paediatric endocrinology   2. Endocrine
    glands—Diseases—Diagnosis
    I. Title
    618.92′40′75   RJ418

ISBN 0–7236–0719–2

Typeset by
Severntype Repro Services Ltd,
The Abbey Business Park, Kingswood, Wotton-under-Edge, Glos.

Printed in Great Britain by
Courier International Ltd, Tiptree, Essex

PREFACE TO REVISED REPRINT

Barely three years after it was first launched, this Handbook appears in a revised reprint to complement the publication of an initial trio (Nephrology, Haematology, Neurology) in a planned series of Handbooks to guide general paediatricians in the investigation of childhood disorders. Experience has shown that the prime objective of such Handbooks is to continue to ensure children are investigated using appropriate tests to produce the maximum information with a minimum of discomfort.

The majority of the changes in the Handbook are confined to the chapter on the Pituitary, particularly in relation to growth hormone secretion. The widespread availability of commercially prepared growth hormone by recombinant DNA technology means that specialized growth clinics are no longer the sole distributors of this hormone for treatment purposes. The non-specialist will more often be deciding which child should receive growth hormone treatment. It is essential to emphasise again the importance of assessing growth velocity accurately in the first instance before embarking on a programme of investigation.

The case illustrations have been retained in their previous format. They demonstrate best which tests should be performed and how the results are to be interpreted. Progress in clinical investigation and research nowadays cannot avoid the science of molecular biology; this is acknowledged by the inclusion of a brief chapter which describes how samples for DNA are obtained and which endocrine disorders can currently be investigated by this technique. No doubt the approach to the investigation of many genetic endocrine disorders will radically alter as more is learned about the human genome.

I. A. Hughes
1989

CONTENTS

Preface to Revised Reprint   v

List of Abbreviations   ix

Foreword   xi

Chapter 1   **General principles of**   1
            endocrine tests

Chapter 2   **The pituitary**   8

Chapter 3   **The thyroid**   60

Chapter 4   **Calcium, parathyroid, vitamin D**   72

Chapter 5   **The adrenal gland**   83

Chapter 6   **The gonads**   110

Chapter 7   **The endocrine pancreas**   130

Chapter 8   **The molecular biology of**   140
            endocrine disease

Appendix   **Normal values**   142

Index   147

LIST OF ABBREVIATIONS

ACTH	adrenocorticotrophic hormone
ADH	antidiuretic hormone (vasopressin)
BS	blood sugar
Ca	calcium
CAH	congenital adrenal hyperplasia
cAMP	cyclic adenosine monophosphate
Ccr	creatinine clearance
cDNA	complementary DNA
Cp	phosphate clearance
CRF	corticotrophin-releasing factor
CT	computerized tomography
DDAVP	1-diamino-, 8-D-arginine-vasopressin (desmopressin)
1,25-DHCC	1,25-dihydroxyvitamin D
DHEA	dehydroepiandrosterone
DHT	dihydrotestosterone
DNA	deoxyribonucleic acid
dopa	3,4-dihydroxyphenylalanine
dopamine	3,4-dihydroxyphenylethylamine
E_2	oestradiol (estradiol)
EDTA	ethylenediamine tetra-acetic acid
FSH	follicle-stimulating hormone
FT_4	free thyroxine
FT_3	free tri-iodothyronine
GC-MS	gas chromatography–mass spectrometry
GFR	glomerular filtration rate
GH	growth hormone
GHRH (GRF)	growth hormone releasing hormone (growth hormone releasing factor)
GnRH	gonadotrophin-releasing hormone
HbA_1	glycosylated haemoglobin
25-HCC	25-hydroxyvitamin D
HCG	human chorionic gonadotrophin
HLA	human leucocyte antigen
HVA	homovanillic acid

IGF-I	insulin-like growth factor I
ITT	insulin tolerance test
17-KGS	17-ketogenic steroids
17-KS	17-ketosteroids
LATS	long-acting thyroid stimulator
LATS-P	long-acting thyroid-stimulating protector
LH	luteinizing hormone
LHRH	luteinizing hormone-releasing hormone (gonadotrophin-releasing hormone; gonadorelin)
17-OGS	17-oxogenic steroids
N	normal
OGTT	oral glucose tolerance test
17-OHCS	17-hydroxycorticosteroids
17-OHP	17-hydroxyprogesterone (17 OH-progesterone)
17-OS	17-oxogenic steroids
PEI	phosphate excretion index
PIF	prolactin-inhibiting factor (dopamine)
PO_+	phosphate
PRA	plasma renin activity
PRL	prolactin
PTH	parathyroid hormone
RIA	radioimmunoassay
rT_3	reverse tri-iodothyronine
T	testosterone
T_4	thyroxine
T_3	tri-iodothyronine
TBG	thyroxine-binding globulin
TDF	testis determining factor
Tg	thyroglobulin
TMCa	tubular maximum reabsorption of calcium
TMP	tubular maximum reabsorption of phosphate
TRH	thyrotrophin-releasing hormone (protirelin)
TRP	tubular reabsorption of phosphate
TSH	thyroid-stimulating hormone
TSI	thyroid-stimulating immunoglobulin
VMA	vanillylmandelic acid

FOREWORD

Professor **R. Hall**
Professor of Medicine
University of Wales College of Medicine

I am very pleased to write an introduction to this first edition of a *Handbook of Endocrine Tests in Children*. Dr I. A. Hughes is well qualified to produce this book. He graduated at the Welsh National School of Medicine and furthered his endocrine training both in this country and in North America. He gained particular insight into the field of steroid biochemistry during his studies at the Tenovus Institute. He is an acknowledged expert in the field of neonatal endocrinology, particularly in the diagnosis and management of disorders of sexual differentiation.

The subject of endocrine tests is complex and, in some areas, controversial. As new hormones are identified new possibilities in testing emerge. For example, with the availability of growth hormone-releasing factor and corticotrophin-releasing factor we now have the ability to test GH and ACTH release directly. Most new tests are established in adults and their application to children needs close liaison between the paediatrician and the adult endocrinologists. In Cardiff, at the University of Wales College of Medicine, close links exist between the author and a large group of basic and clinical endocrinologists including Dr J. Picton Thomas (adrenal); Dr M. F. Scanlon (neuro-endocrinology), Professor R. Hall, Dr J. Lazarus and Dr A. McGregor (thyroid), Dr S. Woodhead (parathyroid and calcium), and Professor K. Griffiths (steroid biochemistry). It is from these frequent contacts that Dr Hughes' endocrine approach has developed and matured.

The introductory chapter on general principles of endocrine testing in children is invaluable, drawing attention to the precautions that must be taken at all stages. The chapters classified according to the major endocrine glands are a model of clarity, with useful advice on the interpretation of the tests. At the end of each chapter illustrative case reports are provided which highlight the application of the tests.

There is no doubt that this text will prove invaluable to all paediatricians called upon to investigate children with endocrine disorders. It will also be helpful to the adult endocrinologist who, in the absence of a paediatric endocrinologist, is frequently involved in the assessment of children. With the amount and rate of expansion of endocrinology, I am sure that a second edition of this excellent Handbook will not be long delayed.

CHAPTER 1

General Principles of Endocrine Tests

Tests of endocrine function (*see Fig.* 1.1) in children usually require serial blood samples and/or 24-h urine collections following the administration of agents which stimulate or suppress hormone levels. The procedures can be unpleasant and may produce side-effects. Appropriate testing should be performed only after detailed history and physical examination has suggested the presence of a specific endocrine disorder. For example, a short child should be investigated for growth hormone (GH) deficiency only after the clinician has been satisfied that the cause is not due to or associated with low birth weight, parental size, adverse social factors, general systemic disease etc. An accurate record of decreased growth velocity determined preferably over one year should be available before arranging endocrine tests. The suitably constructed growth chart has assumed more importance as the benchmark; the often bewildering array of tests of GH secretion should only serve to supplement the anthropometric information.

RANDOM OR DYNAMIC TESTS

In general, random blood samples for hormone measurements in children are unhelpful. This is in contrast to some adult endocrine disorders, such as acromegaly, hyperprolactinaemia and hyperparathyroidism where random GH, prolactin (PRL) and PTH measurements, respectively, are often diagnostic. Since dynamic endocrine tests in infants and children can be technically difficult, it is imperative that no mistakes are made with patient preparation, sample times and volumes, labelling of tubes and request forms, and transporting samples to the appropriate laboratories. If not, the interpretation of results is made difficult and the child may be subjected unnecessarily to a further unpleasant procedure.

PREPARING THE CHILD

The child should be fasted for most endocrine tests. If the child lives locally, the test can be performed as an out-patient. The older child

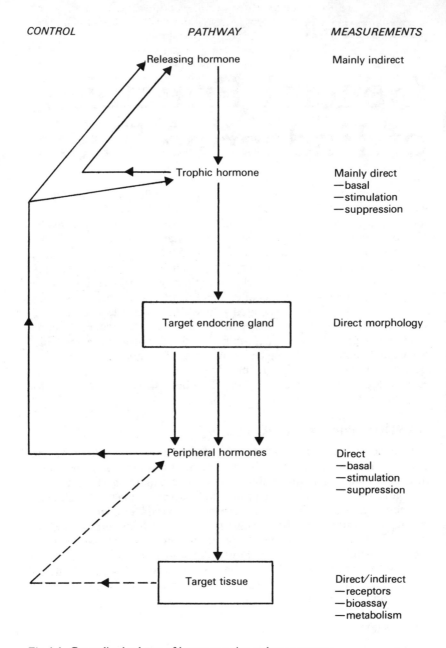

Fig. 1.1. Generalized scheme of hormone action and measurement.

should be fasted (nothing to eat or drink except water) from midnight; this assumes the test will start *no later than* 08:00–09:00. It is unkind, unnecessary and occasionally dangerous to fast a child longer than this. The duration of fasting for infants should not exceed 4–6 hours. If the child is unwell, or is only recently recovering from a systemic illness, the test should be postponed. Ensure that the child has not been receiving any medication or foodstuffs which may interfere with the interpretation of results. Examples include anticonvulsants and thyroid function, iodine-containing compounds or foods (e.g. fish) and radioactive iodine uptake, bananas and urine VMA etc.

COLLECTION OF BLOOD SAMPLES

A reliable intravenous line (i.v.) should be positioned in a large forearm or antecubital vein when sampling blood serially. A 21- or preferably 19-gauge butterfly intermittent infusion set with reseal injection site as an alternative to connecting the i.v. line to a 3-way stopcock allows greater mobility for the child. The infusion line must be maintained patent; this can be achieved using a 20 units/ml solution of heparin–saline (mix 0·2 ml of 1000 units/ml heparin solution with 20 ml saline)* A small volume of blood is withdrawn and discarded before the required venous sample is collected. The infusion set should be adequately 'flushed' through after each sample withdrawal. Careful attention to these details should ensure that the i.v. line functions satisfactorily for the duration of the test.

The improved sensitivity of many hormone assays allows measurement of some hormone concentrations in blood spots. Capillary blood from a finger or heel prick is spotted onto a filter paper disc and allowed to dry. It is important to obtain sufficient blood to completely fill the circle (usually 10 mm diameter) and soak through to the reverse side. For the assay, a standard size smaller disc is punched out and the blood eluded from the paper in a assay tube. Blood spots have the added advantage of allowing more frequent, serial hormone measurements.

Baseline samples must be collected before stimulation and suppression tests are started. Thus, this sample is labelled, $t = 0$ min; if possible an earlier sample $t = -30$ min should also be collected in an attempt to reduce the effect of stress on hormone levels, viz. GH and cortisol. Collect an adequate volume of blood (check with the laboratory) at the required times for each hormone to be measured. Plain (clotted) or heparinized tubes are used depending on whether serum or plasma is the matrix for hormone determination. More than one hormone measurement will usually be determined in each sample. It is advisable to liaise

---

*Pre-mixed solutions are available such as Hep-flush (100 units/ml), Heplok (10 units/ml) and Hepsal (10 units/ml).

with the laboratory staff who normally prefer to aliquot the sample for the different hormone assays *after* the plasma/serum has been separated following centrifugation.

COLLECTION OF URINE SAMPLES

A 24-h urine sample is required for most urinary hormone measurements. Sometimes a fractionated collection, i.e. in 8-h or 12-h aliquots, is required as in the assessment of urine glucose output in diabetic patients. Make certain that the parents or child (if old enough) and *the medical attendants* understand how to collect a 24-h urine sample. The bladder should be emptied and the *time recorded.* This is the *start* of the collection. Each urine voided thereafter for the next 24 hours is collected into a suitable container. At the end of the collection period, the time is recorded on the container. This time signals the start of the next 24-h collection when sequential samples are required. Most urinary hormone measurements do not require the sample to be collected on ice or with a preservative (boric acid or hydrochloric acid) in the container.

Accurate 24-h urine collections in infants and young children are difficult to achieve. Adhesive plastic bags applied around the external genitalia are most commonly used with varying success. Centres where 24-h urine collections are frequently performed may need to design a metabolic crib.[1-3] The creatinine concentration of the urine sample should be determined routinely in order to check the completeness of the 24-h collection.

COLLECTION OF SALIVA SAMPLES

Some endocrine disorders can be investigated by measurement of steroid concentrations in saliva. The advantage of saliva collection over blood or urine sampling is the facility to collect an unlimited number of serial samples by a non-invasive method. The technique is particularly applicable to children. Before sample collection, the mouth should be rinsed with tapwater to remove any food debris. After waiting 1–2 min, whole saliva is collected by gently dribbling into a wide-neck plain tube. Saliva flow can be stimulated by using a drop of citric acid syrup on the tip of the tongue, although this is seldom required. In general, hormone levels in saliva reflect the free hormone concentration in blood.

LABELLING AND PROCESSING OF SAMPLES

This is the time when most mistakes occur. The child's name, hospital number, ward and date of test must be recorded on each sample tube. For dynamic tests (i.e. stimulation and suppression), the time must be *clearly* recorded (i.e. $t = 0, 15, 30, 60, 90, 120$ min etc.). Laboratory request forms must be completed in full, again with the emphasis on name, date and times when samples were collected.

Most laboratories require a separate request form for each hormone determination, particularly if more than one laboratory is involved in the hormone assays. This may create a large amount of paperwork, so it is wise to spend time completing the request forms before starting the test. Pertinent clinical details to be recorded include the child's age, sex and likely diagnosis. The information can help the laboratory staff who may wish to modify the hormone assay in order to obtain maximum information of value to the clinician.

When the test is finished, samples must be transported to the appropriate laboratory without delay. If necessary the investigator should transport the samples personally. This is another link in the chain which can go wrong, particularly in large hospitals. Sometimes blood samples need to be collected on ice, and the plasma/serum prepared immediately using a refrigerated centrifuge, e.g. plasma renin, ACTH. Close liaison with the laboratory staff is essential to ensure satisfactory processing of samples. It is usually the responsibility of the laboratory staff to make arrangements to transport plasma/serum/urine samples to the laboratories in other centres if specialized assays are indicated. There are several systems available for dispatching samples around the country and overseas. Some guarantee next day delivery in the UK. Staff should familiarise themselves with the various options available. It is also a wise precaution to telephone the receiving laboratory to tell staff to expect a sample to arrive. Laboratory staff do not normally take too kindly to evening or weekend arrival times!

The same precautions regarding labelling applies to 24-h urine samples. Either the total volume can be 'recorded on the ward (accurately) and an aliquot (50–100 ml) sent to the laboratory or the entire volume transported to the laboratory. The request form should contain details of the time and date for the start/finish of the collection, in addition to relevant clinical information.

HORMONE ASSAYS

It is beyond the scope of this Handbook to discuss the methods of hormone measurement. Nevertheless, the clinician should have some understanding of the principles involved and limitations imposed on accuracy, reproducibility and speed of 'turn around' in producing results.

Most protein and steroid hormone concentrations, particularly in blood, are currently determined by immunoassay procedures. The procedure involves an analysis of the competition in binding between the hormone in plasma (unknown quantity) and a known quantity of enzyme or radiolabelled hormone, and an antibody specifically directed against the hormone in question. Using a known set of standard concentrations of the hormone, the unknown concentrations of hormone in plasma can be derived from a displacement curve. In some assays, the antibody is radiolabelled. There are several variables in the assay procedure, so that the precision does not always compare favourably with other routine analyses in clinical chemistry. Laboratories who regularly perform immunoassays for hormone measurements participate in both internal and external quality control schemes. If there is 15 per cent variance or more in a result of a sample analysed twice in two separate assays, then it becomes difficult to interpret the absolute value of a single estimation. For example if GH deficiency is defined as a peak serum GH level < 20 mU/l following stimulation, does a value of 18·6, which when repeated is 21·4, constitute GH deficiency? Obviously not. The entire GH profile obtained during a stimulation test must be considered in addition to the clinical findings. In general, results of a laboratory test serve to confirm or refute a diagnosis suggested by clinical examination. Hormone assays are no exception.

NORMAL RANGES FOR HORMONE CONCENTRATIONS

Each laboratory should determine its own range of normal values for hormone concentrations. However, this either may not be available for, or not possible to obtain in, children and young infants. The Appendix contains some data of normal values obtained from the literature; each test protocol is followed by a note on the interpretation of results.

The contents of this chapter may appear pedantic to the reader. However, it cannot be overemphasized that attention must be paid to the following check list when performing endocrine tests in children.

PATIENT PREPARATION

Is there an indication to perform the appropriate endocrine test based on detailed clinical evaluation?

Is the child adequately prepared?—Fasting
                                            —Clinically well
                                            —Any interfering foodstuffs or medications.

Has the height and weight of the child been measured on the day of the test?

Has the dose of the stimulatory/suppressive agent been calculated correctly? (NB. INSULIN DOSE for insulin tolerance test.) IF IN DOUBT, *ASK.*

SAMPLE COLLECTION

Blood
> Secure a reliable i.v. line for serial blood sampling
> Collect basal samples ($t = -30$, 0 min)
> Ensure correct sample tubes—Plain (clotted)
>   —Heparinized.

Urine
> Make sure child/parent and *you* understand how to collect a 24-h urine sample. Is there a suitable container?
> Does it require a preservative?

SAMPLE PROCESSING

Blood tubes/urine containers to be labelled with:
> Name of patient
> Ward/clinic
> Hospital number
> Date of sample
> Time of sample (start and finish for 24-h urine)
> Volume of 24-h urine sample.

Laboratory request forms:
> Write LEGIBLY
> Name of patient
> Age
> Sex
> Ward/clinic
> Hospital number
> Date of test
> Time of sample (start and finish of 24-h urine)
> Test required
> Clinical details of relevance.

Transporting samples:
> Ensure rapid transport to appropriate laboratory
> If necessary contact laboratory staff initially
> If in doubt, transport sample PERSONALLY.

References

1. Winter J. S. D., Baker L. and Eberlein W. R. (1967) A metabolic crib for infants. *Am. J. Dis. Child.* **114,** 150–51.
2. Lewis H. (1977) A cot for metabolic studies. *Arch. Dis. Child.* **52,** 737–8.
3. Lund R. J., Valman H. B. and Platt A. (1980) Device for continuous urine collection in the newborn. *Arch. Dis. Child.* **56,** 880–82.

CHAPTER 2

The Pituitary

The anterior pituitary gland secretes several hormones—GH, TSH, ACTH, PRL, LH and FSH—whose synthesis and secretion are controlled by hypothalamic releasing or inhibiting factors. Some of these factors have been isolated, characterized and synthesised and are used in the evaluation of anterior pituitary function. They include TRH and LHRH. Indirect methods of stimulation are normally used to test the secretory reserve of GH and ACTH. However, releasing factors for these two hormones, GHRH and CRF, respectively, have recently been isolated and characterized. Their use in diagnostic tests is now being evaluated but CRF appears to have little practical application in the investigation of paediatric endocrine disease.

ADH is synthesized in the hypothalamus, transported along axons in the neurohypophyseal tract and stored in the posterior pituitary gland. Secretion from the posterior pituitary is regulated mainly by changes in osmolality of the extracellular fluid. ADH release is assessed by indirect methods.

GROWTH HORMONE

Tests of GH secretion are classified into physiological and pharmacological. The former takes advantage of some normal physiological variables such as exercise and sleep where GH secretion is enhanced.

STIMULATION

Physiological

Random

Occasionally a random blood sample will detect an elevated GH level, particularly if the child is stressed or is fasted.

Such a result would exclude GH deficiency. However, the test is so unreliable that it is not recommended.

There as been a recent resurgance of interest in urinary GH measurements now that more sensitive GH assays are available. A 24 h or an overnight urine collection without preservatives is required. It is preferable to keep the urine stored at $4\,^{\circ}C$ until the collection is completed. An ultrasensitive GH assay is required to detect the low levels associated with GH deficiency. The reliability of using urinary GH assays to screen short children for GH deficiency is currently being evaluated.

Insulin-like growth factor I (IGF-I) is GH-dependent and, as expected, the serum levels of this peptide are low in GH deficiency. Random measurements are too nonspecific for diagnostic use as levels are low in young children and are also affected by liver disease and hypothyroidism. Elevated GH and decreased IGF-I levels are characteristic of Laron's dwarfism.

Exercise

This test should be performed using a bicycle ergometer to generate a standard amount of work which will vary according to the age and size of the child.

One should aim for a physical exertion between 150 and 300 kilopond. m/min equivalent to about 50 per cent maximal working capacity.

    Child fasted

    Blood sample at $t = -30$ and 0 min

    Exercise and bicycle for 10 min ($t = 10$ min)

    Collect blood samples at $t = 10$ and 20 min.

If a bicycle ergometer is not available, the following exercise test is sometimes useful to perform:

    Child fasted

    Blood sample at $t = 0$ min

    Run up and down stairs for 20 min

    Child should be tired, but not exhausted; heart rate should not exceed 180/min

●   Blood sample at end of exercise ($t = 20$ min)

    Rest for 20 min; repeat blood sample ($t = 40$ min).

    Interpretation: A GH level > 15 mU/l excludes GH deficiency. Lower values do not necessarily indicate GH deficiency. If necessary proceed to pharmacological tests. About 20 per cent of exercise-induced tests give false positive results for GH deficiency. Some protocols suggest priming the child with propanolol orally 0·5 mg/kg (maximum dose 40 mg) 1 hour before the test to enhance the GH response. *This carries a risk of hypoglycaemia.*

Sleep

Ideally this test should be performed with EEG monitoring if available.

- Insert i.v. line before bedtime
- Collect 2 blood samples 20 min apart while child awake
- Collect 2 blood samples 20 min apart between stages III and IV
- If no EEG recording, collect 2 samples 20 min apart between 30 and 90 min after onset of sleep.

> *Interpretation:* GH levels during waking hours usually low; the rise in nocturnal levels occurs during stage III and IV sleep equivalent to slow wave sleep. Values > 15 mU/l exclude GH deficiency.
>
> The pulsatile release of GH during a 12–24 h period is studied mainly as part of research protocols. The frequency of blood sampling is usually every 15–20 min and the GH profile is analysed in relation to pulse frequency and amplitude, the integrated concentration of GH during the study period and the area under the curve of the GH profile. Computer programs are available for these detailed analyses.

Pharmacological

Children with short stature and delayed puberty should be primed with sex hormones just prior to the GH stimulation test. The criterion is based on bone age. In delayed puberty and a bone age 10 years or less (determined by Tanner–Whitehouse method) boys are given one dose of Sustanon* 100 mg i.m. 3–5 days before the test; girls are given ethinyl oestradiol 100 µg orally each day for 3 days prior to the test.

Insulin-induced Hypoglycaemia (Insulin Tolerance Test, ITT)

Stress resulting from hypoglycaemia is the stimulus for GH release, believed to be mediated via an α-adrenergic pathway. The dangers are obvious. Contra-indications to performing this test include a history of convulsions, previous hypoglycaemic episodes, and diabetes mellitus.

During an ITT, the following are measured—blood glucose, GH, cortisol and PRL.

- Child must be fasted
- Arrange with laboratory for immediate analysis of blood glucose levels; also monitor capillary blood glucose values using suitable glucose oxidase reagent strips and a glucose meter

---

*A mixture of propionate, phenylpropionate, isocaproate and decanoate esters of testosterone.

- Establish *reliable* i.v. line
- Draw up 20 ml of 50 per cent dextrose solution in a syringe *ready for use*
- Prepare bolus dose of short-acting insulin (Actrapid); usual dose is 0·1–0·15 U/kg body weight. Reduce to 0·05 U/kg if pituitary insufficiency (particularly ACTH deficiency) is strongly suspected
- Collect baseline samples at $t = -30$ and 0 min for blood glucose, GH, cortisol, PRL
- At $t = 0$ min, inject insulin bolus i.v.
- Collect samples at $t = 15, 30, 45, 60, 90, 120$ min for blood glucose and GH
- Collect samples at $t = 30, 60, 120$ for cortisol and PRL.

Symptoms of *hypoglycaemia* usually occur 15–30 min after the insulin injection. If severe, collect an immediate blood sample for hormone analysis, then give i.v. dextrose. At the end of the test, give the child a glucose-containing drink and a meal. DO NOT allow home until observations are satisfactory.

Interpretation: The blood glucose should decrease by 50 per cent or more of the basal value ($t = 0$ min) and/or there should be symptoms and signs of hypoglycaemia—drowsiness, sweating, headache (occasionally nausea and vomiting). With adequate hypoglycaemia, peak GH levels < 7 mU/l indicate GH deficiency. This is excluded with peak GH levels > 15 mU/l. Levels between 7–15 mU/l may indicate partial GH deficiency, but this requires confirmation with a second, different test of GH secretion.

Arginine Stimulation

This has now largely replaced the oral Bovril test. The results are more predictable and reliable. Arginine monohydrochloride (12·5 per cent solution) is infused intravenously over a 30-min period. When infused slowly, side-effects are minimal except for occasional nausea and some irritation at the infusion site.

- Child fasting
- Collect baseline blood sample for GH ($t = -30, 0$ min)
- Start arginine infusion ($t = 0$ min). Infuse 0·5 g/kg body weight over 30 min
- Collect samples for GH at $t = 30, 60, 90$ min.
  Interpretation: GH levels as for ITT.

Glucagon Stimulation

This test is particularly useful in young infants in whom a reliable i.v. line may be difficult to achieve, and in any child where an ITT is contraindicated. Some protocols suggest giving propanolol 0·5 mg/kg orally 2 hours before the test to enhance GH secretion. This may cause hypoglycaemia and bradycardia. An alternative cardioselective β-blocker, betaxolol, is recommended to be a safer adjunct. The dose is 0·25 mg/kg orally.

- Child fasting
- Collect baseline samples for blood glucose and GH ($t = -30$, 0 min)
- At $t = 0$ min, inject glucagon 0·5 mg i.m.
- Collect samples at $t = 30, 60, 90, 120, 180$ min for blood glucose and GH

 Interpretation: GH levels as for ITT. Blood glucose levels should increase two–three-fold above basal value. Glucagon also stimulates insulin release; this is a useful test of pancreatic β cell reserve.

L-Dopa

This is liable to cause nausea and vomiting, particularly in children. Despite this, many investigators favour its use as a reliable and safe screening test for GH deficiency.

Dosage, given orally, is dependent on body weight:

    125 mg—up to 14 kg body weight
    250 mg—up to 32 kg
    500 mg—more than 32 kg.

- Child fasting
- Collect baseline samples for GH ($t = -30$, 0 min)
- Give L-dopa orally
- Collect samples for GH at $t = 30, 60, 90$ min.

 Interpretation: GH levels as for ITT. Propanolol pretreatment (0·5 mg/kg) given orally 2 hours before the test will enhance GH secretion. This may cause hypoglycaemia.

Clonidine Stimulation

This has recently been introduced as a safer test for GH release and produces results as reliable as ITT. Side-effects include drowsiness during the test and a moderate fall in blood pressure which may persist for some hours.

- Child fasting
- Collect baseline samples for GH, cortisol ($t = -30$, 0 min)
- Give clonidine 0·15 mg/m² orally
- Collect samples for GH, cortisol at $t = 30, 60, 90, 120, 150$ min.

 Interpretation: GH levels as for ITT.

Metoclopramide Stimulation

This dopamine antagonist has been shown to release GH in hypogonadal men but not in normal men. The boy with short stature and delayed puberty is functionally hypogonadal. Approximately 70 per cent of such boys release GH following metoclopramide stimulation.

This obviates the need to prime with sex steroids before the test (*see* ITT).

Extrapyramidal reactions such as severe agitation or dystonic movements may occur. Diphenhydramine abolishes the symptoms within minutes.

- Child fasting
- Collect baseline samples for GH, TSH, PRL and cortisol ($t = -30, 0$ min)
- Give metoclopramide 10 mg i.v.
- Collect samples for GH, TSH, PRL and cortisol at $t = 15, 30, 60, 90, 120$ min.

  Interpretation: GH levels as for previous tests. There is also a significant increase in TSH and PRL levels.

GHRH Stimulation (Growth Hormone-releasing Hormone or GRF)

Synthetic GRF is now available, either as 1–40, 1–44 or 1–29 amino acid residue. No significant side-effects have been reported so far, apart from transient facial flushing.

- Child fasting
- Collect baseline sample for GH ($t = -30, 0$ min)
- Give synthetic GRF 1–2 μg/kg i.v.
- Collect samples for GH at $t = 15, 30, 60, 90, 120$ min.

  Interpretation: The peak GH response in normals is highly variable. The test is not reliable, therefore, to make a definitive diagnosis of GH deficiency. However, when used in conjunction with other tests of GH release (e.g. ITT), the results may indicate a hypothalamic rather than a primary pituitary cause for the GH deficiency.

SUPPRESSION

A suppressive test of GH secretion is required if autonomous GH hypersecretion is suspected. Pituitary gigantism or juvenile acromegaly is extremely rare. The GH response to an oral glucose load is assessed.

- Child fasting
- Collect baseline samples for blood glucose, GH and insulin ($t = -30, 0$ min)
- Give glucose 1·75 g/kg orally (maximum 100 g)

- Collect samples for blood glucose, GH and insulin at 0·5, 1, 2, 3, 4, 5 h.

  Interpretation: GH suppresses to undetectable levels in normals. High basal GH levels which fail to suppress and sometimes a paradoxical rise in GH levels is characteristic of GH hypersecretion. There may be evidence of hyperinsulinaemia. In acromegaly there is often an exaggerated GH response to TRH stimulation (*see* later for protocol).

  GHRH testing is of little diagnostic value in juvenile acromegaly.

THYROID STIMULATING HORMONE

Basal levels of TSH are usually low (less than 5 mU/l) in the euthyroid state. More sensitive TSH assays can now detect suppressed TSH levels basally. TSH secretion is under the control of a tripeptide hypothalamic releasing factor—thyrotrophin-releasing hormone (TRH).

TSH Stimulation

Side-effects include nausea and occasional vomiting, particularly if TRH is injected rapidly. Facial flushing and an urge to micturate have been reported.

- It is not essential to fast the child
- Collect baseline samples for TSH, T_4, T_3 (or free T_4 and free T_3), PRL ($t = -30$, 0 min)
- Give TRH 200 μg or 7 μg/kg i.v. over a few minutes
- Collect samples for TSH, PRL at $t = 0, 30, 60, 120$ min and T_4, T_3 (or FT_4, FT_3) at $t = 120$ min.

  Interpretation: Peak TSH levels ranging from 10 to 30 mU/l occur at 30 min. Elevated basal, and exaggerated peak TSH levels are consistent with primary hypothyroidism. Hyperthyroidism (e.g. Graves' disease) is typically associated with suppressed TSH levels unresponsive to TRH stimulation. An exaggerated delayed peak TSH response is suggestive of hypothalamic hypothyroidism, but the distinction from normal is not always clearcut. The TSH response to TRH may be impaired in acromegaly or pituitary gigantism (very rare condition) and in patients receiving suppressive doses of glucocorticoids.

PROLACTIN

In contrast to adults, hyperprolactinaemia rarely occurs in children. However, measurement of PRL is a useful index of hypothalamic-pituitary function. PRL secretion is under tonic inhibition by PIF, produced in the hypothalamus and secreted into the pituitary portal vessels to reach the anterior pituitary gland.

Stimuli for the release of PRL include:

● Stress—hypoglycaemia in ITT
● TRH
● Metoclopramide.

Certain drugs such as the phenothiazines and benzodiazepines, and oestrogens may cause elevated basal PRL levels.

ADRENOCORTICOTROPHIN

The secretion of ACTH is under the control of the hypothalamic decapeptide corticotrophin-releasing factor (CRF). This has been isolated, characterized and synthesized. It is available for limited use in clinical investigation. In general, ACTH secretion is assessed indirectly by measuring the cortisol response to hypoglycaemia and the 11-deoxycortisol response to metyrapone inhibition of cortisol production.

STIMULATION

Insulin Tolerance Test

The protocol is documented in p. 10. The insulin dose should be reduced (0·05 unit/kg) if ACTH deficiency is suspected.

> *Interpretation:* Plasma cortisol levels should rise two–three-fold above basal values in response to adequate hypoglycaemia.

Metyrapone Test

The drug inhibits 11 β-hydroxylase activity in the adrenal cortex leading to reduced cortisol production. This results in increased ACTH secretion and elevated 11-deoxycortisol levels. The steroid can either be measured directly in plasma, or indirectly as urinary metabolites.

Standard Metyrapone Test

● Collect 24-h urine for 17-OHCS or 17-OGS (Day 1)

- Collect 24-h urine sample. Give metyrapone 3.0 g/m^2 orally in 6 divided doses every 4 h starting at 08:00 (Day 2). (An alternative dose regimen is to give 500 mg every 4 hours for body weight $>$ 15 kg; 250 mg every 4 hours for $<$ 15 kg)
- Continue 24-h urine collection and complete metyrapone administration. Collect blood 4 hours after last metyrapone dose for plasma cortisol and 11-deoxycortisol (Day 3)
- Post-metyrapone 24-h urine collection (Day 4).

    Interpretation: Urinary steroid excretion should increase at least two-fold above baseline values. Plasma concentrations of cortisol and 11-deoxycortisol following metyrapone should significantly decrease and increase, respectively. Absent responses occur in ACTH deficiency and following prolonged suppressive glucocorticoid therapy. The response to metyrapone may be inadequate even when an adequate response to ITT has been obtained. An exaggerated response following metyrapone occurs in pituitary-dependent Cushing's syndrome, hypothyroidism and diabetes mellitus.

Short Metyrapone Test

This test relies on the effect of an overnight oral dose of metyrapone to suppress cortisol synthesis. The response may be impaired because of poor absorption of the drug.

- Collect sample at 08:00 hours for plasma cortisol and 11-deoxycortisol (baseline)
- Give metyrapone 30 mg/kg orally at 24:00 hours with a milk drink and snack (to minimize slight nausea)
- Next morning collect sample at 08:00 hours for plasma cortisol and 11-deoxycortisol.

    Interpretation: The morning plasma cortisol level on the second day should be suppressed, with a concomitant increase in plasma 11-deoxycortisol level. Because of the slight risk of acute adrenal insufficiency during the night if ACTH deficiency is present, a modification of this test is to give the oral dose of metyrapone at 08:00–09:00 hours and collect a blood sample 3 hours later to assess the response.

SUPPRESSION

The standard suppression test for ACTH secretion is performed using dexamethasone. There are three tests available.

Overnight Dexamethasone Suppression

● Collect sample of blood (and/or saliva) at 23:00–24:00 hours for cortisol
● Give dexamethasone 1 mg orally at 23:00–24:00 hours
● Repeat sample collection at 08:00 hours.

Interpretation: Midnight cortisol levels are normally low; following a single oral dose of dexamethasone, cortisol levels at 08:00 hours should also be suppressed. This is a screening test and is particularly useful in the child with simple exogenous obesity in whom Cushing's syndrome is suspected. An absence of cortisol suppression requires a more prolonged dexamethasone suppression test.

Low-dose Dexamethasone

● Collect 24-h urine for 17-OHCS and urinary free cortisol; collect blood sample at 08:00 and 24:00 h for plasma cortisol (Day 1)
● Give dexamethasone 5 μg/kg every 6 h for 2 days (Days 2 and 3)
● Collect 24-h urine for 17-OHCS and urinary free cortisol; collect blood at 08:00 and 24:00 hours for plasma cortisol (Day 4).

Interpretation: The urinary steroid excretion should be related to creatinine concentration. Occasionally it may be necessary to administer dexamethasone for 3 days. Failure to suppress confirms Cushing's syndrome (i.e. hypercortisolism) but does not necessarily provide information about the cause.

High-dose Dexamethasone

The protocol is the same as outlined above except that 2 mg dexamethasone is given every 6 hours orally for 2 days.

In older children (> 10 years), the standard low-dose (2 mg daily) and high dose (8 mg daily) dexamethasone dosages for adults can be used.

Note: Another protocol occasionally used is to give dexamethasone 1 mg i.v. every hour for 5 hours with measurements of plasma cortisol at 0 and 6 hours.

GONADOTROPHIN-RELEASING HORMONE

This hypothalamic releasing hormone, a decapeptide, stimulates the release of LH and to lesser extent FSH. The test is usually performed in association with an assessment of gonadal function (*see* later).

- It is not essential to fast the child
- Collect baseline blood samples for LH, FSH, oestradiol (girls), testosterone (boys) ($t = -30, 0$ min)
- Give 100 μg LHRH i.v. or 2·5 μg/kg i.v.
- Collect blood samples at $t = 30, 60, 90, 120$ min for LH, FSH and at $t = 120$ min for oestradiol (or testosterone).

    Interpretation: This depends on the stage of puberty. The prepubertal child shows a small increment in LH and FSH up to 3–4 U/l and 2–3 U/l, respectively. The magnitude of response is greater in early and mid-puberty, particularly for LH. An absent response suggests gonadotrophin deficiency, but this is unreliable in prepuberty and in the child with simple delayed puberty. An exaggerated response, particularly with elevated basal levels, is obtained in precocious puberty (i.e. exaggerated for age) and in primary gonadal failure (e.g. Turner's syndrome).

    The pulsatile release of LH and FSH measured for a 12-hour period overnight is used for research purposes. Serial blood samples must be collected every 20–30 min.

ANTIDIURETIC HORMONE

This hormone is an octapeptide which is synthesized in the hypothalamus, but transported to and stored in the posterior pituitary. Since ADH secretion is controlled mainly by plasma osmolality (and indirectly serum sodium), water deprivation is the main stimulus for testing adequate ADH secretion.

Water Deprivation Test

- Weigh the child
- Collect baseline blood sample for plasma sodium, osmolality, ADH (if available) and urine for osmolality and specific gravity ($t = 0$ h)
- Start fluid fast. NB In children it is seldom necessary to fast longer than 12–16 h (infants no more than 6–8 h)
- Repeat blood and urine samples after 8 h ($t = 8$ h); weigh the child

- Continue until 12–16 h, or as long as tolerated. Weigh the child. Repeat blood and urine samples at 12, 16 h. If no evidence of urinary concentration, give DDAVP 5 μg intranasally or 0·3 μg i.m.
- Collect next available voided urine and a simultaneous blood sample for plasma sodium and osmolality, urine specific gravity and osmolality.

  Interpretation: Plasma osmolality (P) does not exceed 295 mosmol/kg H_2O and urine osmolality (U) increases three-fold to at least 750 mosmol/kg H_2O in normals (or $U/P > 2·0$). Failure to concentrate the urine and P greater than 300 indicates diabetes insipidus. If there is a response to DDAVP, the cause is due to pituitary ADH deficiency. In children, the commonest problem to differentiate is (habit forming) compulsive water drinking. In this situation there is usually urinary concentration following water deprivation. Failure to concentrate and no response to DDAVP indicates nephrogenic diabetes insipidus. Definitive tests of renal function are indicated.

  If assays are available to measure ADH directly in plasma and/or urine, the diagnosis of nephrogenic diabetes insipidus can be established by plotting the urine osmolality against ADH concentration. A shift to the right indicates the higher ADH concentrations required in an attempt to concentrate urine. The analysis can also detect the carriers of this X-linked disorder.

COMBINED TEST OF ANTERIOR AND POSTERIOR PITUITARY FUNCTION

Sometimes called the triple stimulation test, this assesses, using a single protocol, the pituitary hormones previously described. The author's practice is to give the following:

Insulin 0·1–0·15 U/kg i.v.

TRH 200 μg i.v.

LHRH 100 μg i.v.

Collect samples as described in appropriate protocols, followed by:

Arginine 0·5 g/kg i.v.

Sample for GH as per protocol.

Since the child is fasted for the test, a baseline plasma and urine osmolality is usually sufficient to exclude diabetes insipidus.

The chart (*see Fig.* 2.1) summarizes which hormone is measured at each sampling time.

Date of test:

Patient's weight: Height:

Insulin dose:

TRH dose:

LHRH dose:

Starting time:

Additional test:

dose:

Adverse reactions:

Signature of doctor:

Hospital number:

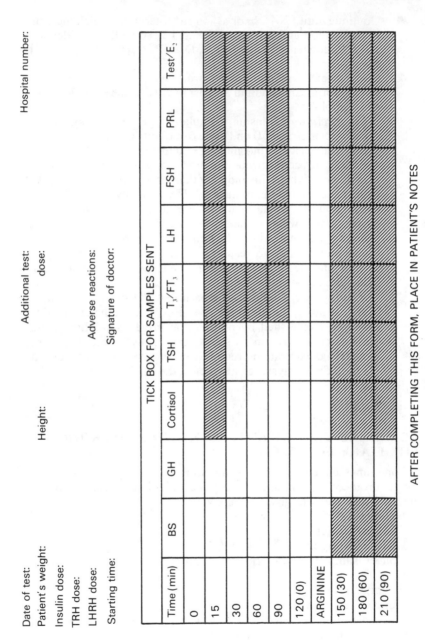

TICK BOX FOR SAMPLES SENT

Time (min)	BS	GH	Cortisol	TSH	T_3/FT_3	LH	FSH	PRL	Test/E_2
0									
15									
30									
60									
90									
120 (0)									
ARGININE									
150 (30)									
180 (60)									
210 (90)									

AFTER COMPLETING THIS FORM, PLACE IN PATIENT'S NOTES

Fig. 2.1. Summary chart for triple and arginine stimulation tests.

THE SHORT CHILD WITH POSSIBLE GH DEFICIENCY

A SUGGESTED METHOD OF INVESTIGATION

Measure height and sitting height accurately
Bone age and height prediction, skull radiograph
General tests —blood count
                  —urea and electrolytes
                  —urinalysis
Repeat measurements 6–12 months later
Repeat bone age and height prediction
Calculate growth velocity; if below 10 th centile for age, perform specific investigations

- Triple stimulation test
Arginine stimulation test
GRF stimulation test
12–24 h GH profile if facilities available
Peripheral karyotype in girls

Decision to start GH
Initial 6 month trial of GH treatment
Dose: 0·5–0·7 units/kg/week in daily divided doses.

CASE ILLUSTRATIONS

1. Delayed puberty (male)
2. Delayed puberty (male)
3. Delayed puberty (male)
4. Delayed puberty (male)
5. Delayed puberty (male)
6. Delayed puberty (female)
7. Isolated GH deficiency
8. Delayed puberty
   Partial GH deficiency
9. Congenital hypopituitarism
10. Panhypopituitarism
    Septo-optic dysplasia
11. GH deficiency (temporary)
    secondary to hydrocephalus
12. Craniopharyngioma
    Panhypopituitarism
13. Nasal rhabdomyosarcoma
    Partial GH deficiency
    (radiation-induced)

14. Pineal-germinoma
    Radiation-induced
      GH deficiency
      gonadotrophin deficiency
15. Medulloblastoma
    Radiation-induced
      hypothalamic damage
      primary ovarian failure
16. Hypogonadotrophic hypogonadism
    Anosmia
    (Kallmann's syndrome)
17. Idiopathic precocious puberty
    (female)
18. Central diabetes insipidus
    Head injury
19. Extreme short stature (non-endocrine cause)
    Ring Y-chromosome anomaly

1. DIAGNOSIS: DELAYED PUBERTY (MALE)

CASE HISTORY

A boy presented with short stature and delayed puberty. At age 13·3 years, height was 139·3 cm ($-$ 2·16 s.d.). He was prepubertal—pubic hair Tanner stage 1 and testes measured 3 ml in volume bilaterally. The bone age determined by the TW2 method was 10·6 years.

INVESTIGATIONS

- Triple stimulation test
    - Insulin 0·15 U/kg i.v.
    - TRH 200 μg i.v.
    - LHRH 100 μg i.v.
- Arginine stimulation
    - 0·5 g/kg i.v.

The patient was primed with androgens (Sustanon 100 mg i.m.) 4 days before the test.

COMMENTS

As expected, low GH and prepubertal LH/FSH values were observed basally. Thyroid function was normal. This must be established before assessing any test of GH release.

Adequate hypoglycaemia was achieved (BS < 2·2 mmol/l and > 50 per cent fall in basal value) and there were also symptoms and signs of hypoglycaemia. A normal peak GH level was obtained at 60 min following insulin and again after arginine stimulation. There was a two-fold increase in cortisol levels thus excluding ACTH deficiency. A normal peak TSH response to TRH stimulation occurred at 30 min. This produced a significant increase in FT_3 indicating normal thyroid responsiveness to this trophic hormone. There was a pubertal peak LH response to LHRH stimulation. The elevated plasma testosterone level was the result of Sustanon priming; this also serves as a useful check that the injection was given.

The results exclude GH deficiency as a cause of short stature. Pituitary function is normal. The gonadotrophin response suggests that the boy will soon develop clinical signs of puberty and a subsequent growth spurt.

RESULTS

Time min	BS mmol/l	GH mU/l	Cortisol nmol/l	TSH mU/l	PRL mU/l
Triple					
0	5·2	4·9	212	1·3	377
15	3·8	2·7	—	—	—
30	1·9	2·0	192	7·9	569
60	4·1	24·0	362	5·6	547
90	5·0	16·6	485	3·8	—
120	5·2	5·4	300	2·5	404

Time min	LH U/l	FSH U/l	FT_4 pmol/l	FT_3 pmol/l	Test nmol/l	E_2 pmol/l
Triple						
0	0·8	0·6	16	8·3	50·4	37
15	—	—				
30	23·1	3·4				
60	19·7	3·3				
90	—	—				
120	11·0	2·3	18	11	37·2	37

● Arginine stimulation

Time min	GH mU/l
0	4·8
30	15·1
60	39·3
90	11·4

2. DIAGNOSIS: DELAYED PUBERTY (MALE)

CASE HISTORY

A boy aged 15·5 years was referred because of short stature and delayed puberty. He was first noticed to be short at age 9 years. Parental heights: father 5'8", mother 5'1". He wanted to join the Army. His height was 145·5 cm ($-3\cdot3$ s.d.). Pubic hair was Tanner stage 2; testes measured 4 ml in volume bilaterally. Bone age was 13·7 years. His height prediction was 162·7 cm, range 157·7–167·7 cm.

INVESTIGATIONS

- Triple stimulation test (Sustanon-primed)
  Insulin 0·15 U/kg i.v.
  TRH 200 μg i.v.
  LHRH 100 μg i.v.
- Arginine stimulation
  0·5 g/kg i.v.

COMMENT

This boy had simple delayed puberty with normal pituitary function. This information and the height prediction were conveyed to the Army Careers Office. He developed puberty spontaneously with a peak height velocity of 11·8 cm/year. His final height is 172·0 cm (25–50th centile) and he has been accepted into the Army.

RESULTS

Time min	BS mmol/l	GH mU/l	Cortisol nmol/l	TSH mU/l	PRL mU/l
Triple					
0	4·9	9·0	240	2·5	313
15	3·2	18·1	—	—	—
30	1·4	31·1	690	5·1	980
60	4·0	24·9	740	4·6	754
90	4·5	13·0	—	—	—
120	4·8	8·5	520	2·5	440

Time min	LH U/l	FSH U/l	T_4 nmol/l	T_3 nmol/l	Test nmol/l
Triple					
0	0·8	0·7	103	2·9	> 30
15	—	—			
30	18·5	3·1			
60	15·5	1·4			
90	—	—			
120	9·9	1·2	112	3·1	> 30

● *Arginine stimulation:*

Time min	GH mU/l
0	8·5
30	> 32
60	> 32
90	13·7

3. DIAGNOSIS: DELAYED PUBERTY (MALE)

CASE HISTORY

Always been short for age. However when the boy started in secondary school, he noticed that he was much shorter than his peers. He was also being teased about his lack of sexual development.

At age 15·1 years, his height was 140·4 cm ($-3·36$ s.d.). He was overweight for his height. Pubic hair was stage 1, but the testes measured 5 ml in volume bilaterally. His bone age was 11·1 years.

INVESTIGATIONS

- Triple stimulation test (Sustanon-primed)
    Insulin 0·15 U/kg i.v.
    TRH 200 μg i.v.
    LHRH 100 μg i.v.
- Arginine stimulation
    0·5 g/kg i.v.
- HCG stimulation
    2000 units i.m. daily for 3 days.

COMMENT

There was no evidence of GH deficiency to account for the short stature. The LH response to LHRH stimulation was exaggerated, especially as he showed only early clinical signs of puberty. There was a very adequate testosterone response to HCG stimulation indicating normal Leydig cell function. He is developing further signs of puberty and is starting a pubertal growth spurt.

RESULTS

Time min	BS mmol/l	GH mU/l	Cortisol nmol/l	TSH mU/l	PRL mU/l
Triple					
0	5·4	0·5	447	1·5	170
15	3·7	5·5	—	—	—
30	2·3	23·4	436	8·8	480
45	2·8	21·6	—	—	—
60	4·8	14·0	475	5·9	330
90	5·2	10·6	—	5·1	300
120	4·6	2·7	259	3·4	190

Time min	LH U/l	FSH U/l	T_4 nmol/l	T_3 nmol/l	Test nmol/l
Triple					
0	0·7	0·6	73	1·8	18
15	—	—			
30	48·8	2·4			
45	—	—			
60	30·7	2·3			
90	—	—			
120	14·8	1·7	93	2·1	22

- *Arginine stimulation:*

Time min	GH mU/l
0	4·0
30	16·0
60	64
90	64

- HCG stimulation:

	Test nmol/l
Pre-	2·4
Post-	31·4

4. DIAGNOSIS: DELAYED PUBERTY (MALE)

CASE HISTORY

Referred at age 17 years because of short stature. His three younger siblings were all taller than him. There was evidence of social deprivation. He was briefly unconscious following a head injury 4 years previously; skull radiograph showed no bone injury. Parental heights; father 5'10", mother 4'11".

Height at 17·4 years was 149·7 cm (− 3·72 s.d.). He was in early puberty (testes measured 4 ml in volume bilaterally). Bone age 14·08 years. Height prediction 158·1 cm; target limits 164·3–181·3 cm.

INVESTIGATIONS

- Sleep GH studies
- Metoclopramide stimulation
     10 mg i.v.
- GHRH stimulation
     100 μg i.v.
- Triple stimulation test (Sustanon-primed)
     Insulin 0·15 U/kg i.v.
     TRH 200 μg i.v.
     LHRH 100 μg i.v.
- Arginine stimulation
     0·5 g/kg i.v.

RESULTS

Time, min	GH mU/l
Sleep study	
Peak—waking	5·9
—sleep	8·2
Metoclopramide	
0	1·6
15	1·2
30	2·2
45	10·4
60	9·1
90	3·4
120	1·9
GHRH	
0	1·7
15	21·0
30	32·6
45	40·0
60	40·0
90	40·0
120	24·6

RESULTS

Time min	BS mmol/l	GH mU/l	Cortisol nmol/l	TSH mU/l	PRL mU/l
Triple					
0	4·6	3·7	63	1·6	147
15	2·1	2·2	—	—	—
30	1·0	1·8	28	6·1	908
60	2·7	32·2	175	5·2	556
90	3·5	15·2	149	4·9	—
120	4·3	8·1	100	4·1	401

Time min	LH U/l	FSH U/l	FT_4 pmol/l	FT_3 pmol/l	Test nmol/l
Triple					
0	1·4	0·7	13	9·2	32
15	—	—			
30	10·5	3·4			
60	5·3	2·8			
90	—	—			
120	5·9	3·0	16	11·4	33

●   Arginine stimulation:

Time min	GH mU/l
0	8·2
30	22·4
60	18·0
90	6·9

COMMENT

This case history illustrates a wide spectrum of results for various GH stimulation tests. Peak GH responses in 3 tests were normal. The cortisol response to profound hypoglycaemia was unusually low. There was an early pubertal gonadotrophin response to LHRH stimulation. At age 18·4 years, height is 152·6 cm and testes measure 8 ml bilaterally. A pubertal growth spurt is imminent.

5. DIAGNOSIS: DELAYED PUBERTY (MALE) PREVIOUS HEAD INJURY

CASE HISTORY

Referred because of short stature. His younger sister was catching him up in height. Had a depressed parietal skull fracture and severe concussion two years previously following a head injury.

His height at age 15·3 years was 146·5 cm (− 2·6 s.d.). He was in early Tanner stage 2 of puberty. His bone age was 12·7 years. A post-exercise GH level was only 2·2 mU/l.

INVESTIGATIONS

- Combined stimulation with (Sustanon-primed)
    Metoclopramide 10 mg i.v.
    TRH 200 μg i.v.
    LHRH 100 μg i.v.
- Arginine stimulation
    0·5 g/kg i.v.
- Fasting plasma and urine osmolality

COMMENT

Insulin-induced hypoglycaemia was not used as a stimulus for GH release in this boy because of a previous severe head injury. Both metoclopramide and arginine produced normal peak GH responses. The gonadotrophin response to LHRH stimulation was pubertal. There were no symptoms of diabetes insipidus and he was able to concentrate his urine after an overnight fast. His growth velocity over the next year was 10·5 cm/year.

RESULTS

Time min	GH mU/l	TSH mU/l	PRL mU/l	LH U/l	FSH U/l	FT$_4$ pmol/l	FT$_3$ pmol/l	Test nmol/l
Metoclopramide/TRH/LHRH								
0	7·9	2·6	128	3·9	1·3	18	8·4	24
15	4·3	—	—	—	—			
30	17·0	9·3	2187	37·7	3·7			
60	10·5	8·1	2719	27·4	4·0			
90	40·0	6·5	—	—	—			
120	39·2	6·3	1337	14·5	3·2	20	13·6	26

● Arginine stimulation:

Time min	GH mU/l
0	39·2
30	64·0
60	63·2
90	31·2

● Fasting osmolality
  Plasma 288 mosmol/kg H_2O
  Urine 940 mosmol/kg H_2O

6. DIAGNOSIS: DELAYED PUBERTY (FEMALE)

CASE HISTORY

Referred for investigation of short stature, delayed puberty and dysmorphic features. Was a full-term infant following a normal pregnancy. She had a *cleft palate.* She had mild hypertelorism, an anti-mongolian slant and short stubby fingers. Previous investigations showed normal calcium, phosphate, alkaline phosphatase, karyotype (46XX), skeletal survey, thyroid function and jejunal biopsy. At age 13·5 years, the peak GH response to insulin-induced hypoglycaemia (BS nadir 1·4 mmol/l) was 6·5 mU/l.

At age 13·9 years her height was 131·0 cm ($-$4·48 s.d.) and sitting height 72·0 cm ($-$4·3 s.d.). Parental heights: father 5'9", mother 5'1". She was prepubertal. Bone age 11·3 years.

INVESTIGATIONS

- Triple stimulation test (Oestrogen-primed)*
  - Insulin 0·15 U/kg i.v.
  - TRH 200 µg i.v.
  - LHRH 100 µg i.v.
- Arginine stimulation
  - 0·5 g/kg i.v.

COMMENT

The possibilities considered in this girl who was extremely short included Turner's syndrome, skeletal dysplasia, pseudohypoparathyroidism and GH deficiency. The latter possibility was strengthened by an association with cleft palate and other mid-line defects. The initial GH response was low, but retesting following oestrogen priming produced a normal GH response both to insulin-induced hypoglycaemia and arginine. Puberty has started spontaneously and there are early signs of a growth spurt. She presumably has genetic short stature in addition to delayed puberty.

---

*Ethinyl oestradiol 100 µg orally each day for 3 days before test.

RESULTS

Time min	BS mmol/l	GH mU/l	Cortisol nmol/l	TSH mU/l	PRL mU/l
Triple					
0	3·7	3·0	815	3·0	150
15	2·7	7·6	—	—	—
30	2·0	18·2	950	7·4	406
60	1·3	6·2	1185	8·2	634
90	1·8	13·3	1174	4·6	—
120	1·8	16·8	1291	4·0	329

Time min	LH U/l	FSH U/l	T_4 nmol/l	Oestradiol pmol/l
Triple				
0	0·8	0·9	112	1200
15	—	—		
30	5·8	3·2		
60	4·2	2·1		
90	—	—		
120	4·4	2·5	124	1250

● Arginine stimulation:

Time min	GH mU/l
0	11·1
30	15·6
60	17·0
90	17·0

7. DIAGNOSIS: ISOLATED GH DEFICIENCY

CASE HISTORY

Presented with short stature at age 4·5 years. Birth weight 3370 g at 40 weeks' gestation. Father 5'3", mother 5'1".

Height 88·0 cm at 4·3 years ($-$ 3·5 s.d.). Growth velocity 4·2 cm/year (< 3rd centile).

INVESTIGATIONS

- Insulin tolerance test
    Insulin 0·15 U/kg i.v.
- Arginine stimulation
    0·5 g/kg i.v.

COMMENTS

The GH response to profound hypoglycaemia was minimal. GH deficiency was subsequently confirmed when GH levels were undetectable following arginine stimulation.

RESULTS

Time min	BS mmol/l	Cortisol nmol/l	GH mU/l
Insulin			
0	4·1	925	1·4
15	4·6	552	0·8
30	1·7	—	3·5
*			
45	11·2	—	—
60	2·3	1035	1·9
90	75·5	—	0·7
120	70·5	940	0·7
Arginine			
0			< 0·5
30			< 0·5
60			< 0·5
90			< 0·5

*Intravenous 50 per cent glucose was given because of severe symptomatic hypoglycaemia.

8. DIAGNOSIS: DELAYED PUBERTY 'PARTIAL' GH DEFICIENCY

CASE HISTORY

Always been shortest child in class at school. Birth weight 5030 g at 40 weeks' gestation. Height of both parents, 5'4". Recent onset of headaches.

Height 119·1 cm at age 10·3 years (− 3·1 s.d.). Prepubertal. Bone age 9·0 years.

INVESTIGATIONS

- Triple stimulation test (a, b)
    - Insulin 0·15 U/kg i.v.
    - TRH 200 μg i.v.
    - LHRH 100 μg i.v.
- Arginine stimulation (a, b)
    - 0·5 g/kg i.v.
- GHRH stimulation
    - 2 μg/kg i.v.

RESULTS

Time min	BS mmol/l		GH mU/l		Cortisol nmol/l		TSH mU/l		PRL mU/l	
Triple	(a)	(b)	(a)	(b)	(a)	(b)	(a)	(b)	(a)	(b)
0	5·2	4·4	3·5	15·0	339	196	2·3	2·2	443	221
15	2·2	1·7	2·2	14·4	—	—	—	—	—	—
30	2·6	1·8	1·3	13·4	535	317	9·9	11·3	1178	563
45	2·4	—	1·2	—	—	—	—	—	—	—
60	2·3	2·3	1·1	15·1	655	466	7·2	8·3	1088	627
90	3·0	2·0	1·6	22·6	602	393	6·0	6·4	900	426
120	2·3	3·3	2·1	23·9	561	363	4·2	4·8	402	354

Time min	LH U/l		FSH U/l		FT_4 nmol/l		FT_3 nmol/l		Test nmol/l	
Triple	(a)	(b)	(a)	(b)	(a)	(b)	(a)	(b)	(a)	(b)
0	<0·8	<0·8	<0·6	<0·6	14	15	8·7	9·1	0·7	0·8
15	—	—	—	—						
30	2·5	2·2	2·1	3·9						
45	—	—	—	—						
60	2·4	2·6	2·7	4·2						
90	2·3	—	2·8	—						
120	2·3	2·2	2·9	6·2	20	22	11·9	12·0	0·6	0·5

- Arginine stimulation
- GHRH stimulation

Time min	GH mU/l	
Arginine	(a)	(b)
0	5·2	15·1
30	5·2	20·1
60	10·5	37·7
90	3·2	28·1
GHRH		
0		21·9
15		46·8
30		50·5
45		57·2
60		56·3
90		50·2
120		44·5

COMMENT

(a)
Despite adequate hypoglycaemia, there was no GH response, but a partial response was obtained with arginine stimulation. The remainder of pituitary function was normal. The gonadotrophin response to LHRH stimulation was appropriate for prepuberty. He was accepted for GH treatment as an idiopathic, isolated GH deficiency. During one year of GH treatment (4 units thrice weekly) his growth velocity was only 4·4 cm/year, equalling the velocity during his pretreatment year. GH therapy was discontinued and he was subsequently re-investigated.

(b)
On this occasion even with elevated basal GH levels, there was a normal peak GH response to each of three different stimuli. Measurement of growth velocity during a one-year trial of GH therapy served as a reliable bio-assay. The discrepant results are difficult to explain, but the case illustrates the need to be wary with making a diagnosis of partial GH deficiency.

9. DIAGNOSIS: CONGENITAL HYPOPITUITARISM

CASE HISTORY

A male infant, birth weight 3990 g, had a hypoglycaemic convulsion 4 hours after a full-term normal delivery. Persistent hypoglycaemia required i.v. glucose initially, followed by frequent high caloric feeds. He was jaundiced and was noted to have a micropenis. There was a normal scrotum containing small testes (< 0.5 ml in volume). Basal GH, cortisol and insulin levels determined when a BS was 1·4 mmol/l were all undetectable. A random TSH was 6·9 mU/l and FT_4 5 pmol/l.

INVESTIGATIONS

- Combined TRH/LHRH stimulation
  TRH 7 μg/kg i.v.
  LHRH 100 μg i.v.
- Glucagon stimulation
  0·5 mg i.m.
- GHRH stimulation
  25 μg i.m.
- Synacthen stimulation
  36 μg/kg i.m.

COMMENT

Hypoglycaemia is unusual in a full-term infant. There was no gestational diabetes or evidence of rhesus haemolytic disease. Plasma insulin was appropriately suppressed when the BS was low, thus excluding hyperinsulinism. Undetectable GH and cortisol levels during hypoglycaemia suggested deficient pituitary production of counter-regulatory hormones. Further clinical evidence for hypopituitarism was the presence of micropenis due to prenatal LH deficiency.

An exaggerated and delayed peak TSH response occurred with TRH stimulation. This is consistent with a hypothalamic defect. An absent gonadotrophin response to acute LHRH stimulation is not unusual in prolonged LHRH deficiency. The explanation for the suboptimal GH response to GHRH and the cortisol response to ACTH is presumably the same. There was no GH response to glucagon stimulation.

Appropriate replacement therapy was started with L-thyroxine and hydrocortisone. Daily GH injections were started to maintain euglycaemia. These were subsequently reduced to thrice weekly injections. Growth velocity has been 29 cm/year during the first 10 months of life. Testosterone therapy will be required for penile growth.

RESULTS

Time min	BS mmol/l	GH mU/l	TSH mU/l	PRL mU/l	LH U/l	FSH U/l	FT₄ pmol/l	FT₃ pmol/l	Test, nmol/l
TRH/LHRH									
0			4·0	80	0·8	0·6	12	2·8	< 0·5
30			6·7	112	0·8	0·6			
60			18·4	145	0·8	0·6			
90			19·3	—	—	—			
120			21·5	146	0·8	0·6	18	4·3	< 0·5
Glucagon									
0	3·4	1·7							
30	6·3	1·6							
60	5·1	2·2							
90	4·2	1·8							
120	1·7	1·1							
GHRH									
0		1·4							
15		3·6							
30		4·3							
45		4·1							
60		4·3							
90		4·3							
120		2·4							

● Synacthen stimulation:

Time min	Cortisol nmol/l	17-OHP nmol/l
0	28	1·0
60	76	1·6

10. DIAGNOSIS: PANHYPOPITUITARISM SEPTO-OPTIC DYSPLASIA

CASE HISTORY

A boy was referred at age 5·5 years for investigation of short stature. He was born at 37 weeks' gestation, birth weight 3200 g. Pregnancy was normal but he was delivered by caesarian section because of an oblique lie. There was perinatal asphyxia and he later developed hypothermia, hypoglycaemia and hyponatraemia. Random plasma cortisol levels were < 50 nmol/l. Treatment was started with cortisone acetate and L-thyroxine. He also developed hydrocephalus which arrested spontaneously.

Height at referral was 92·5 cm (− 3·85 s.d.). Growth velocity during the previous year was 1·7 cm/year. Head circumference was 55 cm (> 97th centile). He had hydrocephalus, low-set ears, truncal obesity and a micropenis. Fundoscopy showed optic nerve dysplasia. The bone age was 3·0 years; his peripheral karyotype was 46 XY.

INVESTIGATIONS

- Arginine stimulation test
    0·5 g/kg i.v.
- Glucagon stimulation test
    0·5 mg i.m.
- Combined TRH/LHRH stimulation tests
    TRH 200 μg i.v.
    LHRH 100 μg i.v.
- Cranial CT scan.

COMMENT

This case illustrates the well-recognized association between septo-optic dysplasia and GH deficiency. The latter is usually part of multiple pituitary hormone deficiencies as in this case. Insulin-induced hypo-glycaemia was not used as a provocative test of GH release in view of the previous neonatal history. Arginine and glucagon stimulation tests were safe and reliable alternatives. Replacement therapy with GH was started; this produced a growth velocity of 11·0 cm/year during the next year. Cortisone acetate and L-thyroxine therapy was continued. The growth of the penis and the potential for spontaneous onset of puberty require assessment later.

RESULTS

Time min	BS mmol/l	GH mU/l
Arginine		
0		< 1·2
30		2·7
60		1·9
90		2·1
Glucagon		
0	4·6	1·5
15	6·9	< 1·2
30	7·1	< 1·2
45	4·0	< 1·2
60	3·6	< 1·2
90	3·3	< 1·2
120	4·6	< 1·2

Combined TRH/LHRH stimulation test

Time min	TSH mU/l	LH U/l	FSH U/l	T_4 nmol/l	T_3 nmol/l
TRH/LHRH					
0	< 0·5	0·8	0·7	118	1·6
30	< 0·5	0·8	0·7		
60	< 0·5	0·8	0·7		
90	< 0·5	0·8	0·7	119	2·1

Cranial CT Scan

This showed gross hydrocephalus. The septum pellucidum was absent.

11. DIAGNOSIS: GH DEFICIENCY (TEMPORARY) SECONDARY TO HYDROCEPHALUS

CASE HISTORY

A boy aged 13 years was referred for investigation of an unsteady gait. His vision had also deteriorated. He had apparently not grown for the previous two years. His height was 155·0 cm (−0·22 s.d.). Head circumference was 97th centile. The visual acuity was reduced and there was bilateral papilloedema. He had severe ataxia. A cranial CT scan showed gross hydrocephalus involving both lateral ventricles and the 3rd ventricle. There was no evidence of a pituitary tumour, but the posterior part of the pituitary fossa was eroded by pressure from the anterior end of the 3rd ventricle.

INVESTIGATIONS (ENDOCRINE)

● Triple stimulation test
Insulin 0·15 U/kg i.v.
TRH 200 μg i.v.
LHRH 100 μg i.v.

RESULTS

Time min	BS mmol/l	GH mU/l	Cortisol nmol/l	TSH mU/l	PRL mU/l
Triple					
0	5·0	0·7	227	2·5	168
15	1·9	1·5	—	—	—
30	2·0	1·8	355	8·4	681
60	4·6	0·7	360	5·6	496
90	4·9	1·8	310	3·9	—
120	5·5	1·2	281	381	187

Time min	LH U/l	FSH U/l	T_4 nmol/l	T_3 nmol/l	Test nmol/l
Triple					
0	1·7	2·4	91	1·8	3
15	—	—			
30	3·2	4·8			
60	3·4	5·4			
90	—	—			
120	2·9	3·9	94	2·1	5

COMMENT

The results indicate complete GH deficiency. The other modalities of anterior pituitary function appear normal. A Spitz–Holter valve was inserted to relieve the hydrocephalus, thought to be secondary to an aqueduct stenosis. There was an improvement in his neurological signs. During the next two years he grew normally and developed puberty spontaneously. Pituitary function was re-evaluated at age 15·3 years:

- Triple stimulation test
    - Insulin 0·15 U/kg i.v.
    - TRH 200 μg i.v.
    - LHRH 100 μg i.v.
- Arginine stimulation
    - 0·5 g/kg i.v.

RESULTS

Time min	BS mmol/l	GH mU/l	Cortisol nmol/l	TSH mU/l	PRL mU/l
Triple					
0	5·3	3·4	326	1·5	102
15	3·9	3·2	—	—	—
30	1·9	1·5	277	4·9	748
45	2·8	13·0	—	—	—
60	3·2	23·6	487	4·8	628
90	2·6	21·4	537	—	—
120	3·6	18·7	306	1·5	254

Time min	LH U/l	FSH U/l	FT₄ pmol/l	FT₃ pmol/l	Test nmol/l
Triple					
0	8·7	4·9	10	3·9	18·1
15	—	—			
30	24·1	7·2			
45	—	—			
60	23·4	8·0			
90	—	—			
120	17·6	6·9	12	5·4	18·8

● *Arginine stimulation:*

Time min	GH mU/l
0	7·2
30	14·0
60	21·6
90	19·1

There was a normal GH response to both insulin-induced hypo-glycaemia and arginine stimulation. Presumably recovery of normal pituitary function occurred following pressure relief from the hydro-cephalus. The gonadotrophin response to LHRH has also changed from prepubertal to a pubertal response.

12. DIAGNOSIS: CRANIOPHARYNGIOMA
PANHYPOPITUITARISM

CASE HISTORY

Deteriorating vision for 2 years. When examined at age 4·8 years, she showed a marked decrease in visual acuity and bilateral optic atrophy. A skull radiograph showed a large pituitary fossa with marked thinning of the dorsum sellae. There was no calcification. Air encephalography performed at that time showed a large pituitary tumour extending above the fossa and almost obliterating the anterior end of the 3rd ventricle. Necrotic tumour was excised at surgery; the histology confirmed a craniopharyngioma.

Height at age 4·8 years was 108 cm (+0·17 s.d.). Growth velocity during the next year was 3·0 cm/year; height at age 5·8 years was 111·0 cm (−0·47 s.d.)

INVESTIGATIONS

● Triple stimulation test
Insulin 0·1 U/kg i.v. (repeat dose 0·15 U/kg)
TRH 7 μg/kg i.v.
LHRH 100 μg i.v.

RESULTS

Basal thyroid function tests 3 months following surgery:
   T_4 12 nmol/l
   TSH < 2·5 mU/l

0·1 mg L-thyroxine was started; T_4 was 178 nmol/l at the time of investigation.

RESULTS

Time min	BS mmol/l	GH mU/l	Cortisol nmol/l	TSH mU/l	LH U/l	FSH U/l	T_4 nmol/l
Triple							
0	4·1	2·1	90	2·5	1·2	< 0·7	170
15	4·1	2·2	112	—	—	—	
30	3·0	2·3	100	2·6	1·5	< 0·7	
45	3·0	3·3	74	—	—	—	
60	3·9	4·3	72	3·1	1·7	< 0·7	
90	4·4	2·8	84	3·2	1·5	< 0·7	168
Insulin 0·15 U/kg							
0	4·0	2·4	80				
15	2·3	4·3	84				
30	2·0	3·4	92				
45	2·9	3·5	117				
60	3·2	2·4	66				

COMMENT

No tests of endocrine function were performed before surgery; it is likely from the extent of the tumour that pituitary dysfunction would have been present at this time. She was hypothyroid post-operatively. No definitive tests of pituitary function were performed until euthyroidism was established with adequate thyroxine replacement. A lower dose of insulin was used in anticipation of ACTH deficiency. This did not produce adequate hypoglycaemia or symptoms thereof. When a 50 per cent fall in BS was achieved with an increased dose of insulin, there was no GH or cortisol response. Absent TSH and gonadotrophin responses to releasing hormones and the presence of diabetes insipidus confirmed panhypopituitarism.

Replacement therapy with thyroxine, hydrocortisone, DDAVP and GH was given. Her growth velocity increased to 8·0 cm/year during the first year of treatment. She will also require oestrogen replacement at an appropriate age.

13. DIAGNOSIS: NASAL RHABDOMYOSARCOMA
PARTIAL GH DEFICIENCY
(RADIATION-INDUCED)

CASE HISTORY

A boy developed a spontaneous haemorrhage from the left ear and a facial palsy at age 7 years. Investigations showed rhabdomyosarcoma of the nasopharynx. He was treated with surgical excision, chemotherapy and radiotherapy. The field of irradiation included the pituitary gland.

Height was 149·8 cm at age 15·1 years ($-2·2$ s.d.). Bone age was 14·2 years. He was in puberty stage 2.

INVESTIGATIONS

- Triple stimulation test (Sustanon-primed)
  Insulin 0·15 U/kg i.v.
  TRH 200 μg i.v.
  LHRH 100 μg i.v.
- Metoclopramide stimulation
  10 mg i.v.

COMMENT

There is evidence of partial GH deficiency following either insulin-induced hypoglycaemia or metoclopramide stimulation. The remainder of pituitary function appears normal. Elevated plasma testosterone levels result from Sustanon priming. During the first year of GH treatment, growth velocity increased from 3·1 to 8·3 cm/year. The boy is continuing pubertal development spontaneously.

RESULTS

Time min	BS mmol/l	GH mU/l	Cortisol mmol/l	TSH mU/l	PRL mU/l
Triple					
0	4·6	12·0	402	2·7	211
15	1·5	7·5	—	—	—
30	2·2	5·8	404	11·7	1096
45	2·9	4·1	—	—	—
60	2·2	4·9	475	8·0	—
90	2·7	10·4	546	5·4	517
120	3·4	11·9	448	4·5	490

Time min	LH U/l	FSH U/l	T_4 nmol/l	T_3 nmol/l	Test nmol/l
Triple					
0	1·0	0·7	111	2·1	> 26
15	—	—			
30	9·9	1·4			
45	—	—			
60	7·8	1·5			
90	3·4	1·4			
120	—	—	105	3·2	> 26

● Metoclopramide stimulation

Time min	GH mU/l
0	1·7
15	3·3
30	5·3
45	—
60	2·8
90	1·8
120	1·9

14. DIAGNOSIS: PINEAL-GERMINOMA
GH DEFICIENCY
GONADOTROPHIN DEFICIENCY
(RADIATION-INDUCED)

CASE HISTORY

Presented at age 9·3 years with occipital headaches, decreased vision, papilloedema, and cerebellar signs. Cranial CT scan showed a mass projecting into the posterior aspect of the 3rd ventricle. The appearance was suggestive of a pinealoma. This was partially removed at surgery. Post-operative radiotherapy and chemotherapy were given.

At presentation his height was 137·0 cm (+0·49 s.d.). By 12·3 years his height was 140·8 cm (−1·27 s.d.) and his growth velocity was 1·7 cm/year.

INVESTIGATIONS

- Triple stimulation test
    - Insulin 0·1 U/kg i.v.
    - TRH 200 μg i.v.
    - LHRH 100 μg i.v.
- Arginine stimulation
    - 0·5 g/kg i.v.

RESULTS

Time min	BS mmol/l	GH mU/l	Cortisol nmol/l	TSH mU/l	PRL mU/l	LH U/l	FSH U/l	FT₄ nmol/l	Test nmol/l
Triple									
0	3·9	1·8	174	3·1	1514	0·6	0·6	78	1·2
15	1·1	1·5	—	—	—	—	—		
30	1·6	1·1	403	10·2	2736	0·7	0·6		
60	1·8	1·2	617	11·7	2430	0·7	0·6		
90	2·3	1·5	527	13·6	2243	—	—		
120	2·7	1·8	564	13·6	1946	0·7	0·6	72	1·1

●   *Arginine stimulation:*

Time min	GH mU/l
0	0·5
30	0·5
60	3·0
90	1·0

COMMENT

There is complete GH deficiency based on two separate stimulatory tests. Gonadotrophin deficiency is probably also present, although the levels are often low in prepuberty. The TSH and PRL (high basal and peak levels) response to TRH are abnormal and suggest radiation-induced hypothalamic damage. Unfortunately the child died from the primary disorder before GH replacement therapy was started.

15. DIAGNOSIS: MEDULLOBLASTOMA
(RADIATION-INDUCED)

Hypothalamic damage
Primary ovarian failure

CASE HISTORY

Partial removal of posterior fossa medulloblastoma at 10 years. Given craniospinal irradiation and chemotherapy. Decreased growth velocity which persisted while in remission and healthy.

Height 131·7 cm at 13·2 years ($-3·4$ s.d.). Growth velocity only 1·2 cm/year. Prepubertal. Bone age 10·1 years.

INVESTIGATIONS

- Triple stimulation test
  Insulin 0·15 U/kg i.v.
  TRH 200 μg i.v.
  LHRH 100 μg i.v.
- Arginine stimulation
  0·5 g/kg i.v.

COMMENTS

There is a partial GH response to arginine stimulation. The basal TSH level is slightly elevated and the peak response is exaggerated. This is probably the result of hypothalamic damage from irradiation, but spinal irradiation may also have produced primary thyroid dysfunction. It has certainly caused primary ovarian failure as shown by elevated basal gonadotrophin levels, increased peak response to LHRH stimulation and low levels of plasma oestradiol. Thyroxine, GH and oestrogen replacement is required.

RESULTS

Time min	BS mmol/l	GH mU/l	Cortisol nmol/l	TSH mU/l	PRL mU/l
Triple					
0	3·8	6·1	128	5·1	297
15	2·3	5·4	—	—	—
30	1·3	3·5	254	40	1730
45	1·6	3·6	—	—	—
60	2·2	2·8	557	38	1560
90	2·4	3·3	—	—	—
120	2·6	1·9	550	20	900

Time min	LH U/l	FSH U/l	T_4 nmol/l	T_3 nmol/l	E_2 pmol/l
Triple					
0	11·2	24·4	73	1·5	60
15	—	—			
30	> 40	> 50			
45	—	—			
60	> 40	> 50			
90	—	—			
120	> 40	> 50	72	2·1	71

● Arginine stimulation

Time min	GH mU/l
0	1·8
30	4·3
60	11·3
90	1·9

16. DIAGNOSIS:
HYPOGONADOTROPHIC HYPOGONADISM
ANOSMIA
(Kallmann's syndrome)

CASE HISTORY

Referred at age 13·0 years with micropenis and delayed puberty. He was a forceps delivery, birth weight 3660 g. He developed hydrocephalus which arrested spontaneously at age 2 years. Bilateral orchidopexy was performed at age 10 years because of undescended testes. He was always 'accident prone' and clumsy, and was in a remedial class at school. He had anosmia (absent sense of smell). Both testes were descended but measured only 1·5 ml in volume. The penis was small (stretched length < 2·5 s.d.).

INVESTIGATIONS AND RESULTS

- Peripheral karyotype 46 XY
- LHRH stimulation
  100 μg i.v.
- Short HCG stimulation test
  2000 units i.m. daily for 3 days
- Long-term HCG stimulation test
  2000 units i.m. twice weekly for 3 weeks

LHRH stimulation

Time min	LH U/l	FSH U/l	Testosterone nmol/l
0	1·8	1·0	2·3
30	2·4	0·2	
60	2·3	0·3	
120	2·2	0·4	2·1

HCG stimulation

	Testosterone nmol/l
Short	
Pre	2·1
Post	2·0
Long-term	
Pre	2·0
Post	2·8

COMMENT

The combination of isolated gonadotrophin deficiency and an olfactory defect is termed Kallmann's syndrome. This resulted in bilateral cryptorchidism and micropenis. The growth of the penis is dependent on normal fetal LH secretion during the latter part of gestation. An absent plasma testosterone response to a short HCG stimulation test is compatible with prolonged gonadotrophin deficiency. However, the inadequate response following longer-term HCG stimulation suggests possible primary gonadal damage also. Treatment was started with Sustanon 100 mg i.m. each month. The growth of the penis has been satisfactory. As expected, the testes remain small.

This boy has two uncles with Kallmann's syndrome. They are currently receiving a trial of therapy with pulsatile long-acting LHRH analogue.

17. DIAGNOSIS: IDIOPATHIC PRECOCIOUS PUBERTY (FEMALE)

CASE HISTORY

Referred at age 4·2 years because of early signs of puberty. The mother had been concerned about breast development 1–2 years previously but had been reassured that it was only fatty tissue. She was noted to be tall at age 2 years. Pubic hair and a vaginal discharge had developed recently, but no menses. She was advanced for her age, preferring to mix with 7–8-year-old children. Height was 118·2 cm (+4·1 s.d.). Breast development and pubic hair were stages 4 and 3, respectively. The remainder of the physical examination was normal.

INVESTIGATIONS AND RESULTS

- Bone age 10·4 years
- Cranial CT scan *normal*
- Pelvic ultrasound
  Increased size of uterus for age
  No ovarian cysts
- Serum T_4 120 nmol/l
  TSH 2·3 mU/l
  PRL 146 mU/l
- LHRH stimulation
  100 μg i.v.

LHRH stimulation

Time min	LH U/l	FSH U/l	Oestradiol pmol/l
0	2·0	3·4	220
30	> 50	17·3	—
60	> 50	16·4	—
120	38·6	14·1	240

COMMENT

This girl had true precocious puberty. Onset of menses was imminent. The cause was central, i.e. premature activation of the hypothalamic-pituitary–ovarian axis. No intracranial lesion was demonstrable. Treatment was initially started with cyproterone acetate. During the next six months her growth velocity was 10·6 cm/year and bone age advanced 1 year. Treatment was changed to an LHRH long-acting analogue (D-Ser (TBU)^6—LHRH-EA^{10}; Buserelin, Hoechst) given intranasally. One month later, peak LH and FSH responses to acute LHRH stimulation were 8·7 U/l and 3·0 U/l, respectively.

18. DIAGNOSIS: CENTRAL DIABETES INSIPIDUS HEAD INJURY

CASE HISTORY

A boy aged 14 years fell off his bicycle and injured his head. He lost consciousness only momentarily but vomited for the next 24 h. A right 6th nerve palsy was noticed at this time. He subsequently became excessively thirsty, passed large volumes of urine frequently and developed nocturnal enuresis. When examined, there were no abnormal physical signs and the cranial nerve palsy had resolved. A cranial CT scan was normal.

INVESTIGATIONS AND RESULTS

● Water deprivation test

Fast	Weight	Plasma		Urine	U/P Ratio
		Na	Osmolality	Osmolality	
h	kg	mmol/l	mosmol/kg H_2O	mosmol/kg H_2O	
0	43·3	141	287	72	
6	43·0	143	308	102	
10	42·1	144	298	124	
12	41·6	147	299	175	0·6
DDAVP 20 μg intranasally					
13		147	299	314	
15		144	280	514	
16		140	275	898	3·3

Note: Weight loss during 12-h water deprivation was 4·3 per cent body weight
12-h overnight urine output *before* DDAVP = 2500 ml
12-h overnight urine output *after* DDAVP = 450 ml

● Triple stimulation test
Insulin 0·15 U/kg i.v.
TRH 200 μg i.v.
LHRH 100 μg i.v.

RESULTS

Triple stimulation test

Time min	BS mmol/l	GH mU/l	Cortisol nmol/l	TSH mU/l	PRL mU/l
0	5·1	7·2	155	2·6	128
15	3·2	16·2	—	—	—
30	1·1	13·1	133	14·9	415
60	4·9	19·6	133	11·3	321
90	4·4	7·5	104	9·5	—
120	4·8	4·7	129	7·3	177

Time min	LH U/l	FSH U/l	FT_4 pmol/l	FT_3 pmol/l	Test nmol/l
0	3·5	1·9	16	7·9	20·8
15	—	—			
30	22·0	4·2			
60	18·3	4·1			
90	—	—			
120	14·5	3·8	22	12·2	24·0

COMMENT

This boy had symptoms of polydipsia, polyuria, enuresis and a failure to concentrate urine after 12-h water deprivation. He lost weight significantly. The U/P ratio was low (normal $> 2 \cdot 0$). A central (i.e. pituitary) cause for the diabetes insipidus was confirmed by a normal response to DDAVP (U/P ratio increased to 3·3). Presumably head trauma had caused diabetes insipidus, possibly associated with a fracture of the base of the skull. Anterior pituitary function was not affected, although there was a subnormal cortisol response to hypoglycaemia. Diabetes insipidus is well controlled with twice daily intranasal DDAVP.

19. DIAGNOSIS: EXTREME SHORT STATURE
(non-endocrine cause)
RING Y-CHROMOSOME ANOMALY

CASE HISTORY

Referred at age 14·5 years for investigation of extreme short stature. First noted to be small in early infancy. Was then thin, pot-bellied and had a ravenous appetite. Investigations for 'failure to thrive' were normal. Birth weight 3360 g at 40 weeks gestation.

At age 14·5 years, height was 129·6 cm (− 4·1 s.d.). In early stage 2 puberty. Bone age 12·5 years. Growth velocity measured over 1 year was 2·8 cm/year.

INVESTIGATIONS

- Exercise GH test
- Triple stimulation test (Sustanon-primed)
    - Insulin 0·15 U/kg i.v.
    - TRH 200 μg i.v.
    - LHRH 100 μg i.v.
- Arginine stimulation
    - 0·5 g/kg i.v.
- Sleep GH studies

RESULTS

Time min	BS mmol/l	GH mU/l	Cortisol nmol/l	TSH mU/l	PRL mU/l	LH U/l	FSH U/l	T_4 nmol/l	Test nmol/l
Exercise									
Pre-		1·2							
Post-		6·3							
Triple									
0	4·0	2·4	233	2·5	167	0·7	0·4	101	50
15	1·8	2·3	—	—	—	—	—		
30	1·4	10·8	221	10·5	386	27·0	0·9		
45	2·0	21·7	—	—	—	—	—		
60	2·9	17·5	441	8·7	352	22·8	0·6		
90	3·6	14·4	332	7·5	340	—	—		
120	3·8	13·6	289	6·3	299	13·5	0·6	104	48
Arginine									
0		10·4							
30		24·6							
60		32							
90		32							
Sleep									
Awake		1·3 (peak value)							
Sleep		8·1 (peak value—stage III)							

COMMENT

There was no endocrine cause for the short stature based on these results. Additional investigations performed included:

- Skeletal survey—*No bone dysplasia*
- Jejunal biopsy —*Normal*
- Ba meal   —*Normal*
- *Karyotype*   —Mosaic 45 X/46 X, r(Y)
  No normal Y detected in any of the cells.

The chromosome anomaly consisting of ring formation of the Y-chromosome indicates loss of chromosome material. In this case it explains the reason for extreme short stature. Karyotype analysis is *not* one of the first tests to perform for the investigation of short stature in a boy. However, in the absence of any abnormality detected during extensive endocrine and non-endocrine tests for short stature, a karyotype in this instance provided the answer.

CHAPTER 3

The Thyroid

There are a large number of tests available to assess thyroid function. Functionally they can be divided into:

Thyroid profile—to define a state of euthyroidism, hypothyroidism or hyperthyroidism

Definitive tests of thyroid function to establish aetiology of thyroid disease.

THYROID PROFILE

THYROXINE

This measures total thyroxine (T_4), usually by radioimmunoassay. Serum T_4 is elevated in:

- Hyperthyroidism
- Pregnancy
- In response to oestrogens (e.g. oral contraceptives)
- Familial increased thyroxine-binding globulin (TBG) concentration.

Serum T_4 is decreased in:

- Hypothyroidism
- Severe hypoproteinaemia, e.g. nephrotic syndrome
- Familial decreased TBG concentration.

TRI-IODOTHYRONINE

Total serum tri-iodothyronine (T_3) is increased and decreased in conditions similar to those listed for T_4. The syndrome of T_3 toxicosis (normal T_4, but elevated T_3) is extremely rare in children.

THYROID STIMULATING HORMONE

An essential measurement when T_4/T_3 concentrations are low. In the presence of elevated TSH, this thyroid profile is indicative of primary hypothyroidism.

FREE THYROXINE AND FREE TRI-IODOTHYRONINE

Until recently, these tests were very time-consuming and unavailable for routine use. Using RIA techniques, FT_4 and FT_3 measurements are now widely available and are rapidly replacing total T_4 and T_3 measurements. Their main advantage is the lack of interference with changes in thyroxine binding protein concentrations. Certain drugs and severe, non-thyroid illness can affect free hormone levels.

Other tests of thyroid function available, but not measured routinely include the following.

REVERSE TRI-IODOTHYRONINE

The term 'reverse' refers to the alternative metabolic pathway of T_4 monode iodination; rT_3 is metabolically inactive, but is preferentially increased in the fetus, newborn and in severe, non-thyroid illness. Its measurement has limited use clinically.

THYROXINE BINDING GLOBULIN

The major binding protein for T_4 and T_3 can be measured directly by RIA. Alterations in TBG concentrations have been referred to previously. There is no evidence that a familial increase or decrease in TBG concentration is associated with a particular clinical disorder.

THYROGLOBULIN

Tg is measured by RIA. Since Tg levels should be undetectable in serum in the absence of any thyroid tissue, Tg measurements are useful to monitor treatment of metastatic thyroid cancer, and as an index of the amount of thyroid tissue present in infants with congenital hypo-thyroidism.

In summary, for routine use a thyroid profile requires a random, non-fasting blood sample for:

- TSH
- T_4 or FT_4
- T_3 or FT_3.

DEFINITIVE TESTS

THYROID AUTO-ANTIBODIES

These are present in the serum of patients with auto-immune thyroid disease. Auto-antibodies, most frequently measured by a variety of techniques, include:

- Anti-thyroglobulin
- Anti-microsomal
- Anti-colloid.

Other organ-specific auto-antibodies may also be present in association with thyroid auto-immune disease. These include islet cell auto-antibodies (insulin-dependent diabetes mellitus), adrenal auto-antibodies (Addison's disease) and gastric parietal cell auto-antibodies.

Interpretation: Thyroid auto-antibodies are usually present in high titre (> 1 in 40) in Hashimoto's thyroiditis, occasionally in Graves' disease, and sometimes associated with other auto-immune diseases.

THYROID-STIMULATING IMMUNOGLOBULINS

These are IgG immunoglobulins that bind directly to the thyroid TSH receptor; in most instances they have stimulating properties leading to hyperthyroidism (Graves' disease). Variously termed in the past 'long-acting thyroid stimulator' (LATS) and 'long-acting thyroid stimulating-protector' (LATS-P), the more general term 'thyroid-stimulating immunoglobulins' (TSI) is now applied. Typically, the infant of a mother with Graves' disease may have high levels of TSI at birth which decrease over a period of 6–8 weeks. Neonatal hyperthyroidism can occur. Occasionally the TSH receptor antibody can have an inhibitory effect on thyroid function leading to transient neonatal hypothyroidism. Measurements of TSI are available in certain specialized laboratories.

TSH STIMULATION TEST

This test and the interpretation of results has been discussed in Chapter 2 (p. 14).

RADIOACTIVE ISOTOPES

Thyroid scintigraphy

Isotopes usually used are:
- $^{99}Tc^m$—pertechnetate
- ^{123}I—sodium iodide.

Information obtained from this test includes:

Detection of thyroid tissue, e.g. congenital hypothyroidism

Location of tissue, e.g. ectopic

Definition of extent of a goitre

Establishment of nature of a thyroid nodule, i.e. whether 'hot' or 'cold'.

^{123}I-labelled sodium iodide uptake

This is the preferred isotope for use in children since it is concentrated more in the thyroid gland and the half-life is short.

Less radiation dose is administered if a scintigram is not required.

Dose: Infants < 1 year—0·1 MBq (2·7 μCi) i.v.

Children—dose is a proportion of the adult dose (1 MBq) based on body weight

If a scan is also required, the dose is 10 times greater.

Note: MBq is a megabequerel, an SI unit of measure.

Interpretation: After an oral dose, ^{123}I uptake is usually measured at 4 h; further uptake measurements at 24 and 48 h are sometimes indicated. In Graves' disease, the uptake at 4 h will be elevated (usually more than 40 per cent). If a dyshormonogenesis is suspected, a perchlorate discharge test should be performed.

- Give standard ^{123}I dose orally
- Measure uptake at 1 h
- Give potassium perchlorate orally

    Dose: < 2 y   —100 mg

           2–12 y—200 mg

           > 12 y   —400 mg

Interpretation: If organification is normal, no more than 5–10 per cent of the radioactive iodide is discharged following perchlorate administration. In dyshormonogenesis associated with an organification defect, 60–70 per cent of the accumulated radioactivity is discharged within 1 h. A discharge of radioactive iodide sometimes occurs in Hashimoto's thyroiditis, but not of the same magnitude.

THYROID ULTRASOUND

This is not performed routinely and its reliability in detecting thyroid tissue in congenital hypothyroidism is not clearly established.

SUGGESTED PROTOCOL FOR INVESTIGATION OF CONGENITAL HYPOTHYROIDISM

INFANT

- Blood for TSH, FT_4, FT_3, Tg, CPK, thyroid autoantibodies, bilirubin
- Radiograph left knee for femoral/tibial epiphyses
- ^{123}I scan (plus possible perchlorate discharge)
- Thyroid ultrasound
- Clinical photograph

MOTHER

- Blood for TSH, FT_4, FT_3, thyroid autoantibodies, (plus possibly TSI).

CASE ILLUSTRATIONS

1. Congenital hypothyroidism
   Ectopic sublingual thyroid
2. Congenital hypothyroidism
   False positive creatine kinase test
3. Primary hypothyroidism
   Dyshormonogenesis

4. Primary hypothyroidism
   Auto-immune thyroiditis
5. Auto-immune thyroiditis
   (Hashimoto's)
   Alopecia areata
6. Hyperthyroidism (Graves' disease)

1. DIAGNOSIS: CONGENITAL HYPOTHYROIDISM
ECTOPIC SUBLINGUAL THYROID

CASE HISTORY

Elevated filter-paper blood spot TSH (132 mU/l) detected during routine newborn hypothyroid screening programme. Normal full-term pregnancy, birth weight 3600 g. Infant clinically euthyroid. No goitre palpable.

INVESTIGATIONS AND RESULTS

- Infant serum

TSH	325 mU/l
FT_4	8 pmol/l (N 8–26)
FT_3	5·3 pmol/l (N 3–9)

- Knee radiograph

  Femoral epiphysis present

  Tibial epiphysis present

- ^{123}I scan

  There was uptake only in an area above the hyoid bone; probably sublingual thyroid

- Maternal serum

TSH	1·2 mU/l
FT_4	13 pmol/l
FT_3	5·4 pmol/l

COMMENT

The initial TSH value on screening was clearly elevated. In response to a marked increase in serum TSH, free thyroid hormone concentrations were at the lower end of the normal range determined in *adults*. The scan detected a remnant of thyroid in an ectopic position which was presumably producing sufficient thyroid hormone to maintain euthyroidism *in utero*. There was no evidence of maternal thyroid dysfunction. Replacement therapy was started with L-thyroxine 10 μg/kg per day.

2. DIAGNOSIS: CONGENITAL HYPOTHYROIDISM
FALSE POSITIVE CREATINE KINASE
TEST

CASE HISTORY

A male infant had an elevated filter-paper blood spot TSH (225 mU/l) at age 7 days detected through the routine newborn hypothyroid screening programme. The infant was full-term, birth weight 3250 g. He was clinically euthyroid. There was a strong family history of Duchenne muscular dystrophy.

INVESTIGATIONS AND RESULTS

- Infant serum
    - TSH   775 mU/l
    - FT_4 < 1 pmol/l
    - FT_3 1·1 pmol/l
- Serum creatine kinase 995 IU/l (N 0–130)
- Radiograph knee—femoral and tibial epiphyses absent
- ^{123}I scan–no radio-iodine uptake seen; athyreosis
- Maternal serum
    - TSH   1·5 mU/l
    - FT_4 12·9 pmol/l
    - FT_3 6·0 pmol/l

COMMENT

Congenital hypothyroidism was confirmed by an elevated serum TSH, undetectable free thyroid hormone concentrations and athyreosis on ^{123}I scan. A creatine kinase screen was performed because of the family history. This was markedly elevated. However, after 2 months' treatment with L-thyroxine 10 μg/kg per day, serum creatine kinase concentration had fallen to 169 IU/l (FT_4 23 pmol/l, TSH 53 mU/l). An increase in the concentration of creatine kinase is well recognized in primary hypothyroidism affecting adults. Further studies are required to determine whether this is common in newborn infants with primary hypothyroidism.

3. DIAGNOSIS: PRIMARY HYPOTHYROIDISM DYSHORMONOGENESIS

CASE HISTORY

A boy referred at age 12·0 years because of a goitre. He had cold intolerance and always felt tired. There was some difficulty with swallowing. The family were from Iraq and the parents were not related. A brother apparently had a goitre at birth which disappeared with thyroid extract treatment. The boy had a large diffuse, non-tender goitre. The skin was dry and the peripheries felt cold. He was in early puberty. Bone age was 11·4 years.

INVESTIGATIONS AND RESULTS

● Serum

      T_4 12 nmol/l

      TSH   60 mU/l

● Thyroid auto-antibodies *negative*

● ^{123}I uptake

      61 per cent at 4 h

      38 per cent at 48 h

● ^{123}I uptake and perchlorate discharge

      80 per cent of ^{123}I discharged within 30 min

● Thyroid fine needle biopsy

      No evidence of lymphocytic infiltration

      Findings compatible with a dyshormonogenesis.

COMMENT

This boy's goitre was associated with mild clinical signs of hypothyroidism but profound biochemical evidence of primary hypo-thyroidism. Auto-immune thyroiditis is usually accompanied by positive auto-antibodies, but this is not absolute. There was an increased 4 h uptake of ^{123}I with failure of organification. This may be associated with sensorineural deafness (Pendred's syndrome). An audiogram was normal. The fine needle biopsy of the thyroid also showed no evidence of auto-immune disease. It is possible that the brother has a similar syndrome, inherited as an autosomal recessive. Treatment was started with L-thyroxine 0·1 mg (100 μg) daily. The goitre decreased in size, he became more active and had a growth spurt. After 6 months his serum T_4 and TSH were 95 nmol/l and 8·0 mU/l, respectively.

4. DIAGNOSIS: PRIMARY HYPOTHYROIDISM AUTO-IMMUNE THYROIDITIS

CASE HISTORY

A girl referred at age 8·5 years because of short stature. Previous health normal. Had coarse facial features, short neck, low hairline, short upper arms. She was obese. Height 103·9 cm ($-4·07$ s.d.). Sitting height 57·7 cm ($-3·98$ s.d.).

INVESTIGATIONS AND RESULTS

● Peripheral karyotype —46XX
● Skeletal survey—*normal*
● Bone age—4·0 years
● Urinary mucopolysaccharide screen—*negative*
● Serum
      TSH   52 mU/l
      T_4 12 nmol/l
● Thyroid auto-antibodies
      Thyroglobulin—*positive*
      Microsomal—*positive*
      Colloid—*positive*
● ^{123}I uptake and perchlorate discharge
      4 per cent uptake at 1 h; no evidence of discharge

COMMENT

The clinical signs of hypothyroidism were not obvious in this girl. Turner's syndrome was the most likely diagnosis. The presence of thyroid auto-antibodies, low T_4, elevated TSH confirmed that hypothyroidism was primary and due to auto-immune (Hashimoto's) thyroiditis. Treatment was started with 100 µg L-thyroxine daily. Her growth velocity increased to 9·7 cm/year during the first year of treatment.

5. DIAGNOSIS: AUTO-IMMUNE THYROIDITIS (HASHIMOTO'S). ALOPECIA AREATA

CASE HISTORY

A girl aged 11·5 years presented with a goitre. Her only complaint was tiredness. There was no family history of thyroid disease. Her height was 149·0 cm (+0·39 s.d.). She was prepubertal. There was a firm, nodular, non-tender goitre. She was clinically euthyroid. At this time serum T_4 was 149 nmol/l and TSH < 2·5 mU/l. She was reviewed 3 months later.

INVESTIGATIONS AND RESULTS

- Serum

  T_4 37 nmol/l

  TSH   > 40 mU/l
- Thyroid auto-antibodies

  Thyroglobulin red cell test—*positive* 1/80

  Thyroid microsomal red cell test—*positive* 1/100

  Thyroid colloid immunofluorescence—*positive*

  Thyroid microsome immunofluorescence—*positive*
- Plasma calcitonin 0·11 μg/l (N< 0·08 μg/l)
- ^{123}I uptake 10 per cent at 4 h (N 10–40 per cent)

  Effective thyroxine ratio (ETR) 1·14 (N 0·86–1·13)

COMMENT

Biochemical evidence of hypothyroidism developed within 3 months of initial presentation. Because of a firm nodular goitre, plasma calcitonin was also measured. This was only marginally raised and was normal on subsequent measurements. An auto-immune thyroiditis can cause similar findings on clinical examination. This was confirmed by the presence of thyroid auto-antibodies, a low 4-h ^{123}I uptake and a slightly increased ETR. She has also developed patches of alopecia which were probably auto-immune mediated. She was treated with L-thyroxine 0·1 mg (100 μg) daily. The goitre decreased in size, she developed signs of puberty and had a growth spurt. Her patches of alopecia grew hair again spontaneously. Final height is 170·0 cm (+ 1·3 s.d.) and menses are regular.

6. DIAGNOSIS: HYPERTHYROIDISM
(GRAVES' DISEASE)

CASE HISTORY

A boy aged 8 years was referred because of weight loss despite a voracious appetite. There were no bowel symptoms. His mother stated that he had become very active and temperamental. He was a pre-term infant (34 weeks' gestation) but there were no neonatal problems. A maternal grandmother had a thyroidectomy for hyperthyroidism. His height was 122·0 cm (+ 0·73 s.d.) and weight 20·4 kg (3–10th centile). Heart rate was 110/min, regular, blood pressure 120/60. Both eyes were prominent with a conspicuous stare. There was a mild chemosis and lid retraction. He had a diffuse small goitre which was non-tender. A soft bruit was audible over the gland. There was also an early soft systolic murmur audible at the cardiac apex. He had a fine tremor of the outstretched hands. Bone age was 8·5 years.

INVESTIGATIONS AND RESULTS

Serum

T_4	136 nmol/l
T_3	4·2 nmol/l
TSH	< 1·5 mU/l
Thyopac-3	75 per cent
FT_4I	181 nmol/l
FT_3I	5·5 nmol/l

^{123}I uptake
    55 per cent at 4 h
    70 per cent at 24 h
Thyroid auto-antibodies
    Thyroglobulin red cell test—*positive* 1/320
    Thyroid microsomal red cell test—*positive* 1/100
    Thyroid colloid immunofluorescence—*positive*
    Thyroid microsome immunofluorescence—*positive*
Thyroid-stimulating immunoglobulins—*positive*
    93 per cent inhibition of TSH binding (N< 15 per cent)

TRH stimulation test
    200 μg i.v.

Time min	TSH mU/l	PRL mU/l
0	< 1·5	150
30	1·6	800
60	< 1·5	560
120	< 1·5	420

COMMENT

Hyperthyroidism is uncommon in childhood, particularly in boys. The clinical diagnosis was confirmed by the presence of increased thyroid hormone concentrations and undetectable basal serum TSH. With the improved sensitivity in TSH assays it is possible to differentiate between normal and hyperthyroid states using basal serum TSH measurements. In this case, autonomous hyperthyroidism was confirmed by an absent TSH response to TRH stimulation. Further confirmation was obtained from the increased ^{123}I uptake. Thyroid auto-antibodies were positive and the cause of Graves' disease was confirmed by the presence of thyroid-stimulating immunoglobulins. Treatment was started with carbimazole, 0·75 mg/kg per day (15 mg daily in 3 divided doses). Within 3 months, serum T_4 was 13 nmol/l and TSH $>$ 40 mU/l. He was therefore treated with a 'blocking' regime using a combination of carbimazole and L-thyroxine. His current medication is carbimazole given as 5·0, 2·5 and 2·5 mg every 8 hours and L-thyroxine 0·1 mg daily. He is clinically euthyroid and growing normally.

CHAPTER 4

Calcium, Parathyroid, Vitamin D

This chapter describes the investigations required to determine the causes of *hypo-* or *hypercalcaemia* associated with either parathyroid disease or disordered vitamin D metabolism. It is important to exclude a non-endocrine cause for abnormal calcium metabolism, such as chronic renal failure. Hypocalcaemia is the more frequent problem in children. Neonatal hypocalcaemia is a relatively common transient condition and is not due to a persistent endocrinopathy. Note that, occasionally, neonatal hypocalcaemia is the result of *maternal* hyperparathyroidism; do not forget to check the plasma calcium level in the mother.

HYPOCALCAEMIA

The total plasma calcium must be determined on more than one occasion with the patient *fasted* before more detailed and complex investigations for the cause of hypocalcaemia are started. If possible, the blood sample should be collected with the least amount of venous stasis.

BASAL INVESTIGATIONS
- Collect *fasting* blood sample, preferably between 09:00–10:00 h
- Plasma Calcium
      Phosphate
      Alkaline phosphatase

Total protein and albumin
Creatinine
Electrolytes
● Serum magnesium
● Ionized plasma calcium (not routinely available)
● Serum PTH
● Plasma vitamin D metabolites
  25-Hydroxycholecalciferol (25-HCC)
  1,25-Dihydroxycholecalciferol
  (1,25-DHCC; not routinely available)
● 24-h urine for calcium
  Phosphate
  Creatinine
  Hydroxyproline.

Interpretation: The plasma Ca should always be interpreted in relation to the protein concentration. The following profiles suggest specific diagnostic *possibilities* as the cause for hypocalcaemia:

Ca ↓	PO_4 ↑	PTH low or undetectable	—Hypoparathyroidism
Ca ↓	PO_4 ↑	PTH ↑	—Pseudohypoparathyroidism
Ca N (↓)	PO_4 ↓	Alk. phosphatase ↑	*—Rickets*

Rickets can be classified according to aetiology by additional basal investigations interpreted in the following way:

● Plasma 25-HCC ↓   *Vitamin D deficiency*
  PTH ↑(N)   *Rickets (Nutritional)*
● Plasma 25-HCC N   *Vitamin D-dependent*
  Plasma 1,25–DHCC ↓   *Rickets— Type I*
  Plasma PTH ↑ (N)
● Plasma 25-HCC N   *Vitamin D dependent*
  Plasma 1,25-DIICC (N)   *Rickets— Type II*
  Plasma PTH ↑ (N)
  (receptor defect)
● Plasma 25-HCC N   *Vitamin D-resistant*
  Plasma 1,25-DHCC N   *(Hypophosphataemic)*
  PTH N
  PO_4 ↓↓   *Rickets*

NB: The results of these basal investigations should also be interpreted in relation to a clinical and radiological assessment of the specific cause of rickets. Standard tests of renal function must be performed to exclude a primary renal cause (e.g. chronic renal failure, Fanconi syndromes).

DYNAMIC INVESTIGATIONS

The principal dynamic test for the investigation of hypocalcaemia is an assessment of the renal response to exogenous PTH. The results determine the cause of hypoparathyroidism.

Urinary cAMP and phosphate response to PTH (previously referred to as Ellsworth–Howard test).

- Patient to be fasted except for water allowed *ad libitum*
  Encourage 100–150 ml hourly oral intake throughout the test
- Empty bladder at start of test ($t = 0$ h)
- Collect 2×30 min (0·5 h) urine samples for baseline calcium, phosphate, creatinine and cAMP (time = 0·5, 1·0 h). Urine samples should be acidified and stored at $-20°C$
- Collect blood samples for calcium, phosphate, cAMP and PTH at 0·5 and 1·0 h
  NB Check with laboratory for correct processing of blood sample for cAMP
- Infuse bovine PTH 100–200 units i.v. over 30 min (time 1·0–1·5 h). Bovine PTH should be dissolved in 2·5 ml human albumin solution and made up to 60 ml volume (reduce this volume in infants as appropriate) with normal saline
- Collect 3 × 30 min (0·5 h) urine samples for calcium, phosphate, creatinine and cAMP (time = 1·5, 2·0, 2·5 h)
- Collect blood samples for calcium, phosphate, cAMP and PTH at 1·5 and 2·5 h
- NB The *volume* of each 30-min urine sample must be recorded accurately.
  Interpretation: In normals and patients with hypoparathyroidism, there is a 10–20-fold increase in plasma and urinary cAMP after PTH, and at least a 2-fold increase in urinary phosphate excretion. There is also usually an increase in plasma calcium indicating bone responsiveness to PTH. The phosphate excretion can be expressed in several ways:

a. Ratio of phosphate clearance (Cp) to creatinine clearance (Ccr)

$$\frac{Cp}{Ccr} = \frac{\text{Plasma creatinine} \times \text{Urine phosphate}}{\text{Plasma phosphate} \times \text{Urine creatinine}}$$

b. Percentage tubular reabsorption of phosphate (Percentage TRP)

$$\text{Percentage TRP} = 1 - \frac{Cp}{Ccr} \times 100$$

c. Phosphate excretion index (PEI)

$$\text{PEI} = \frac{Cp}{Ccr} - (0\cdot055) \times (\text{plasma phosphate})$$

d. Tubular maximum reabsorption of phosphate (TMP). A nomogram is available to calculate this value.[1]
e. Ratio of TMP to glomerular filtration rate (TMP/GFR).

In *pseudohypoparathyroidism* there is an absent urinary cAMP and phosphate response to PTH infusion, referred to as 'type I'. Very rarely there is a normal urinary cAMP response but a blunted phosphate response, termed 'type II'.

HYPERCALCAEMIA

This is uncommon in children. Confirmation of hypercalcaemia is essential before embarking on extensive investigations. An elevated *fasting* plasma Ca should be confirmed on *three* separate determinations.

BASAL INVESTIGATION

- Plasma phosphate
- Plasma alkaline phosphatase
- Total protein and albumin
- Plasma creatinine
- Plasma electrolytes (including chloride), pH
- Serum PTH
- 24-h urine for calcium, phosphate, creatinine, hydroxyproline, cAMP.

    Interpretation: A normal or detectable serum PTH level in the presence of hypercalcaemia is inappropriate and indicates hyperparathyroidism. This condition is rare in childhood. Parathyroid hyperplasia rather than adenoma is the usual cause; the plasma calcium can be markedly elevated. Urinary phosphate clearance (as determined by one of the methods shown on pp. 76–77) is typically elevated.

The condition labelled familial hypocalciuric hypercalcaemia is characterized by increased plasma calcium, decreased urinary calcium excretion and usually a normal serum PTH. Other causes of an increased plasma calcium include vitamin D intoxication, sarcoidosis, malignancy and Addison's disease. Apart from the possibility of excessive vitamin D ingestion, these causes of hypercalcaemia are extremely unlikely in childhood. Rarely a glucocorticoid suppression test may be required.

DYNAMIC INVESTIGATIONS

Hydrocortisone Suppression Test

- Collect baseline fasting blood sample for plasma calcium and PTH
- Give hydrocortisone 2 mg/kg per day orally in 8-hourly divided doses for 10 days
- Repeat blood samples for plasma calcium and serum PTH on days 8 and 10.

    Interpretation: Typically there is no suppression of plasma calcium in primary hyperparathyroidism; in contrast the plasma calcium decreases following glucocorticoid administration in vitamin D intoxication, sarcoidosis and malignancy. However, the results may not be clearcut, particularly when hypercalcaemia is associated with a malignant tumour.

Other Dynamic Tests

These include an assessment of the plasma calcium and serum PTH response to
  a. A diuretic
  b. A calcium infusion.
These tests are not recommended since they seldom provide further useful information and are potentially dangerous.

CALCITONIN

Calcitonin is a 32-amino acid polypeptide synthesized and secreted by the parafollicular ('C') cells situated in the thyroid. The hormone is discussed in this chapter since its principle action is to lower plasma calcium concentration. At present there is no recognized disorder due to either an increased or a decreased production of calcitonin except perhaps osteoporosis. However, calcitonin levels are *increased* in meduallary carcinoma of the thyroid. Thus its measurement in plasma serves as a useful diagnostic marker for this tumour, and subsequently as an index of recurrence following treatment.

BASAL INVESTIGATIONS

- Collect fasting blood sample and transfer immediately to a cooled heparinized plastic tube. Separate plasma immediately using a refrigerated centrifuge. A haemolysed specimen invalidates the results.

  Interpretations: In normals, basal plasma calcitonin levels are usually low or undetectable. An elevated basal value suggests medullary carcinoma of the thyroid, although a certain proportion of patients can have a normal basal value. Calcitonin levels can also be elevated with other malignancies (particularly pancreatic endocrine tumours) and in chronic renal failure.

  Since medullary carcinoma of the thyroid is often familial, other members of the family *particularly children*, should be screened. This requires a provocative test of calcitonin secretion.

DYNAMIC INVESTIGATIONS

Pentagastrin Stimulation Test

- Patient to be fasted
- Collect baseline blood sample for plasma calcitonin ($t = 0$ min)
- Inject pentagastrin 0·5 μg/kg body weight i.v. rapidly (over 10–20 s)
- Collect blood samples at $t = 2, 5, 10, 15$ and 20 min for plasma calcitonin
- NB The blood samples for calcitonin determination should be processed as described under 'Basal investigations.'

  Interpretation: An exaggerated plasma calcitonin response following pentagastrin stimulation suggests medullary carcinoma of the thyroid. Absolute values depend on the assay method employed. For example, a peak calcitonin value > 200 pg/ml is abnormal.

Other Stimulation Tests

These include:
- Calcium infusion
- Whisky stimulation test.

The results of these tests are less reliable than those obtained using a pentagastrin stimulation.

NB   Medullary carcinoma of the thyroid may be inherited as part of a *multiple endocrine neoplasia syndrome* (termed 'type II'). Other components of the syndrome include hyperparathyroidism and phaeochromocytoma. The appropriate investigations for these disorders are found in the relevant sections of this Handbook.

References

Walton R. J. and Bijvoet O. L. M. (1975) Nomogram for derivation of renal threshold phosphate concentration. *Lancet,* **ii,** 301–310.

CASE ILLUSTRATIONS

1. Primary hyperparathyroidism
   Parathyroid adenoma
2. Vitamin D resistant (hypophosphataemic) rickets
3. Pseudohypoparathyroidism

1. DIAGNOSIS: PRIMARY HYPERPARATHYROIDISM PARATHYROID ADENOMA

CASE HISTORY

Hypercalcaemia was found in a 15-year-old girl whose father had primary hyperparathyroidism. On direct questioning she had symptoms of polydipsia only. She was normotensive but had corneal calcification.

INVESTIGATIONS AND RESULTS

- Plasma

Calcium	3·17 mmol/l
Phosphate	0·51 mmol/l
Total protein	69 g/l
Albumin	46 g/l
Corrected calcium	3·05 mmol/l
Alkaline phosphatase	376 IU/l

- Serum

Creatinine	70 μmol/l
PTH	1·4 ng/ml

- 24-h urinary

Calcium	8·0 mmol/24 h
Phosphate	18·6 mmol/24 h

- Radiographs of skull and hands *normal*
- Thallium technetium scan
    Increased uptake in left superior part of thyroid
- TMP/GFR   0·5   (N 0·7–1·4 mmol/l)
- TMCa/GFR   2·58 (N 1·6–2·1 mmol/l)

COMMENT

This girl had a calcium screen performed because of the family history of hyperparathyroidism. Serum PTH was inappropriately elevated in the presence of hypercalcaemia. Decreased plasma phosphate and tubular reabsorption, increased tubular reabsorption of calcium and a positive thallium scan all substantiated the diagnosis of primary hyperparathyroidism. There was no evidence of renal dysfunction.

A large left superior parathyroid gland (2·0 × 1·5 cm) was removed at surgery. Three normal, small parathyroid glands were identified. Histology of the excised gland was consistent with a parathyroid adenoma. The following profile was obtained at post-operative review: calcium 2·51, phosphate 1·45, PTH < 0·3.

The details of this case were kindly provided by Mr M. H. Wheeler, Consultant Surgeon, Cardiff.

2. DIAGNOSIS: VITAMIN D RESISTANT (HYPOPHOSPHATAEMIC) RICKETS

CASE HISTORY

A female at age 13 months developed bowing of the legs and a waddling gait. By age 23 months, her height was 76·0 cm (− 3·1 s.d.). She was a full-term infant, birth weight 3150 g. She had been bottle fed and given appropriate multivitamin supplements during her first year of life. Radiographs of the wrists and knees showed evidence of severe rickets.

INVESTIGATIONS AND RESULTS

- Plasma

Calcium	2·54 mmol/l
Phosphate	0·70 mmol/l
Alkaline phosphatase	250 IU/l
Urea	*normal*
Electrolytes	*normal*
Creatinine	*normal*
Blood gases	*normal*
Amino acids	*normal*

- Serum PTH   0·6 ng/ml
- Plasma 25-HCC   18·5 ng/ml
- Urine pH   5·0

COMMENT

The history and results of investigations excluded vitamin D deficiency, chronic renal disease and generalized renal tubular dysfunction as the cause of rickets. Normal slit-lamp ophthalmic examination excluded cystinosis. Plasma phosphate was decreased in keeping with a primary renal tubular defect producing hyper-phosphaturia, hypophosphataemia and rickets. The child was treated with 1 α-hydroxyvitamin D_3 and phosphate supplements. This healed the rickets and improved her linear growth. The disorder is inherited as a sex-linked dominant. It is interesting that, in this case, there were no affected members in the family and the patient was female. Presumably there had been a spontaneous mutation.

The details of this case were kindly provided by Dr H. V. Price, Lecturer in Child Health, Cardiff.

3. DIAGNOSIS: PSEUDO-HYPOPARATHYROIDISM

CASE HISTORY

A girl aged 3 years was referred for investigation of developmental delay. She was the product of a normal pregnancy, birth weight 3400 g. Her initial development was normal. She had an odd facies and was obese. As part of routine investigation, she was noted to be hypocalcaemic (plasma Ca 1·57 mmol/l, PO_4 2·88 mmol/l, alkaline phosphatase 819 IU/l). Treatment was started with vitamin D 3000 units daily. Hypocalcaemia persisted despite increasing the dose of vitamin D to 12000 units daily. She developed recurrent generalized convulsions usually associated with febrile episodes.

INVESTIGATIONS AND RESULTS

- Plasma

Calcium	1·34 mmol/l
Phosphate	2·90 mmol/l
Alkaline phosphatase	294 IU/l
Urea	3·2 mmol/l
Creatinine	34 μmol/l
Total protein	63 g/l
Albumin	38 g/l

- Serum Mg   0·65 mmol/l
- Serum PTH   20 ng/ml
- Radiographs
  - Skull   *normal*
  - Hands   All metacarpals short, but features not diagnostic of pseudohypoparathyroidsm
- Response to exogenous bovine PTH infusion

Time min	Plasma Ca mmol/l	PO$_4$ mmol/l	Urine PO$_4$ mmol/l	cAMP nmol/l	cAMP/creat. ratio	Fractional PO$_4$ excretion
−15	1·35	2·95	—	—	—	—
0	—	—	7·3	1270	0·59	0·03
15	1·36	3·05	—	—	—	—
30	—	—	5·4	670	0·74	0·06
45	1·40	2·94	—	—	—	—
60	—	—	4·5	570	0·95	0·07
75	1·46	2·88	—	—	—	—
90	—	—	1·0	280	0·80	0·07
105	1·42	3·03	—	—	—	—
120	—	—	0·3	260	0·87	0·13

Note: An age-matched control demonstrated an increase in the cAMP/creatinine ratio from 0·67 to 11·07 following an infusion of the same batch of bovine PTH.

COMMENTS

There was no evidence of rickets and hypocalcaemia failed to respond to conventional vitamin D therapy. Renal function was normal; elevated endogenous PTH in the presence of hypocalcaemia suggested a diagnosis of pseudohypoparathyroidism. This was confirmed by an absent plasma calcium, urinary cAMP and urinary phosphate response to exogenous PTH. The latter was shown to be biologically active in a normal control. Occasionally there is a dissociation between the phosphaturic and urinary cAMP responses in pseudohypoparathyroidism; this has been termed 'type II'. Treatment was started with 1 α-hydroxycholecalciferol (alfacalcidol) 1 µg daily. Plasma calcium had returned to normal three months later.

The details of this case were kindly provided by Dr M. Purcell, Consultant Paediatrician, Tameside General Hospital, Ashton-Under-Lyne.

CHAPTER 5

The Adrenal Gland

The adrenal gland is composed of a cortex and medulla whose function and control are completely independent. Tests of function are described separately.

ADRENAL CORTEX

Three classes of steroid hormone are synthesized by the adrenal cortex.

- Glucocorticoids, e.g. cortisol
- Mineralocorticoids, e.g. aldosterone
- Sex steroids—androgens, e.g. dehydroepiandrosterone
  —oestrogens, e.g. oestrone.

The investigator must be familiar with some steroid structures in order to understand the nomenclature of tests to be described later.

The basic steroid nucleus is a four-ring structure containing 17 carbon atoms numbered as follows.

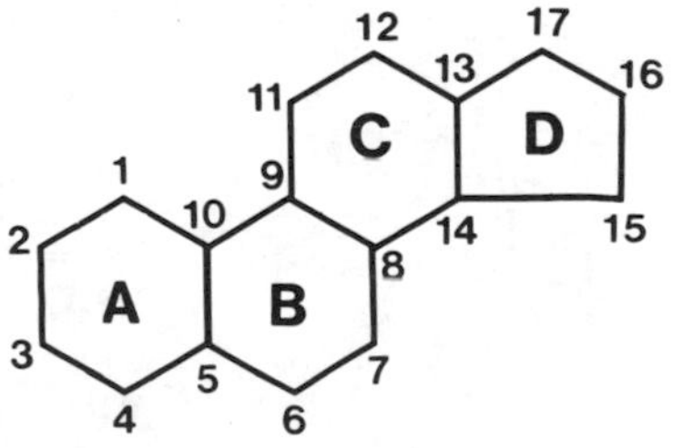

Fig. 5.1. Basic steroid nucleus.

Additional C atoms define the parent compound of the 3 main groups of steroids. Thus:

- C18 steroids—oestrogens
- C19 steroids—androgens
- C21 steroids—glucocorticoids and mineralocorticoids.

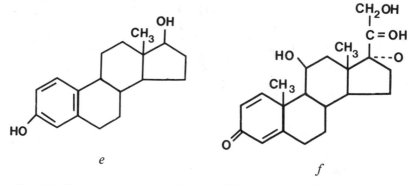

Fig. 5.2. Steroid structures. (*a*) Cortisol; (*b*) progesterone; (*c*) aldosterone; (*d*) testosterone; (*e*) oestradiol; (*f*) prednisolone; (*g*) fludrocortisone; (*h*) dexamethasone.

g   h

The steroid ring structures of some common naturally occurring and synthetic steroids are illustrated in *Fig.* 5.2.

Adrenal steroid biosynthesis proceeds via a series of enzymatic steps starting with cholesterol and is under the control of ACTH (*see Fig.* 5.3). Knowledge of this pathway is essential to interpret tests of adrenal function, particularly when investigating suspected congenital adrenal hyperplasia.

TESTS OF ADRENOCORTICAL FUNCTION (GLUCOCORTICOIDS)

BASAL

Plasma

Cortisol is the predominant steroid produced by the adrenal cortex. There is a pronounced diurnal rhythm in cortisol secretion which is lowest between 18:00 and 02:00 h and at its peak between 04:00 and 10:00 h. The secretion is also episodic. Consequently single random measurements are of limited value.

To assess diurnal rhythm collect blood samples:

- At 09:00 and 24:00 hours (or bedtime)
- Use heparinized tubes
- Sample volumes required are small (1–2 ml) because of high sensitivity of most cortisol assays.

> *Interpretation:* Night-time values of cortisol should be approximately 50 per cent of the early morning value. Stress, particularly if due to a difficult venepuncture, can cause a marked increase in levels. Recent development of assays for cortisol in *saliva* offers a practical solution to this problem,

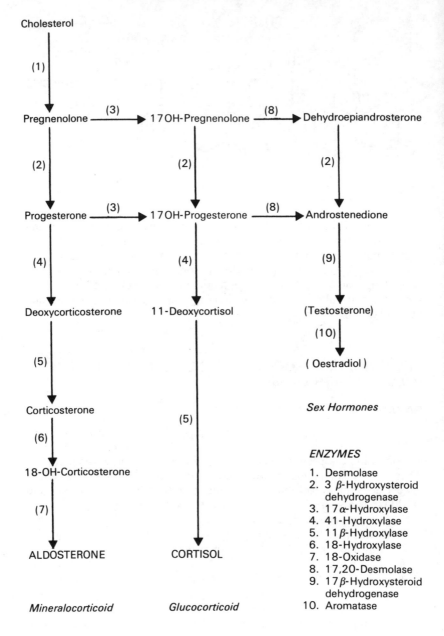

Fig. 5.3. Scheme of adrenal steroid biosynthesis.

particularly in children. Persistently elevated morning and night-time cortisol levels in the absence of stress, is consistent with hypercortisolism and requires further investigation (*see* later).

Other adrenal steroid hormones which can be measured *routinely* in plasma include the following:

- Progesterone
  17-Hydroxyprogesterone
  11-Deoxycortisol
- Aldosterone
  Dehydroepiandrosterone and its sulphate
  Androstenedione
  Testosterone
  Oestradiol.

Most are secreted episodically and display a diurnal pattern. Single measurements may be diagnostic for some inherited disorders of steroid biosynthesis, e.g.

17-Hydroxyprogesterone—congenital adrenal hyperplasia due to 21-hydroxylase deficiency (*see Fig.* 5.3)

11-Deoxycortisol—congenital adrenal hyperplasia due to 11β-hydroxylase deficiency (*see Fig.* 5.3)

Dehydroepiandrosterone—congenital adrenal hyperplasia due to 3β-hydroxysteroid dehydrogenase deficiency.

Many of these steroids can now also be measured in saliva and blood spots.

ACTH

This measurement is not available routinely. Since there is a diurnal rhythm in secretion, measurements should be performed at 09:00 and 24:00 hours simultaneously with plasma cortisol. The blood sample must be collected into cooled heparinized tubes, immediately centrifuged at 4 °C and the plasma stored at − 20 °C until assay. The plasma ACTH/cortisol profile can be very informative.

Interpretation:

- Elevated ACTH, low cortisol—primary adrenal insufficiency; requires Synacthen stimulation test
  Low ACTH, low cortisol—pituitary deficiency and secondary adrenal insufficiency
  Low or undetectable ACTH and hypercortisolism—Cushing's syndrome due to adrenal tumour
  Normal or elevated ACTH and hypercortisolism—pituitary dependent Cushing's syndrome (Cushing's disease)
  Very high ACTH and hypercortisolism—ectopic ACTH syndrome (rare in children).

These basal tests of adrenal function, if abnormal, are followed by stimulation/suppression tests (*see* pp. 91–92).

Urine

Before the development of sensitive assays to measure steroid concentrations in plasma, adrenocortical function was investigated by measurement of urinary glucocorticoid metabolites. In many centres, this continues to be the practice. Creatinine excretion should be measured as an index of the completeness of urine collection.

- *24-h 17-hydroxycorticosteroid (17-OHCS)*
  This is usually measured using a colorimetric method which depends on the presence of a hydroxyl group at carbon positions 17, 21 and a ketone group (oxo, $C = O$) at carbon position C-20 (*see Fig. 5.1*). The test mainly measures urinary metabolites of cortisol, cortisone and 11-deoxycortisol.
  Interpretation: Elevated in Cushing's syndrome: urinary 17-OHCSs are also increased in obesity, pregnancy, hyperthyroidism, renal failure. Certain drugs also interfere with the test. This is not a reliable index of hypercortisolism.

- *24-h urine oxogenic or ketogenic steroids (17-OGS or 17-KGS)*
  This method is based on the measurement of all C21 steroids containing a 17OH group: this is transformed to a ketone-group ($C = O$), i.e. ketosteroids or oxosteroids. Hence the term oxo*genic* or keto*genic*. The oxosteroids 'generated' are measured by the classical Zimmermann reaction. The test mainly measures urinary metabolites of cortisol, cortisone, 11-deoxycortisol and 17OH-progesterone.
  Interpretation: As for 17-OHCS.

- *24-h urinary 17-oxosteroids or ketosteroids (17-OS or 17-KS)*
  This method is based on the presence of an *oxo* (ketone)-group at C-17. The test measures the concentration of weak adrenal androgens such as DHEA and androstenedione, but *not* testosterone (since it has an OH group at C-17). The test is neither a reliable index of cortisol nor of androgen secretion.

- *24-h urinary free cortisol*
  This test measures a fraction (normally less than 1 per cent) of total cortisol secretion which is excreted unchanged. It is a reliable index of hypercortisolism, and is not increased in simple obesity.

- *24-h urinary pregnanetriol*
  This test measures the urinary metabolite of 17OH-progesterone and was used extensively in the diagnosis of congenital adrenal

hyperplasia before the development of plasma steroid radio-
immunoassays. It has now been largely superseded.
NB   Add 10 ml 2 per cent boric acid to the urine container as
a preservative.
● *11-oxygenation index*
   The index is a measure of the ratio of oxygenated to non-
   oxygenated steroids in the C-11 position. Only a random urine
   sample (10–20 ml) is required, which is the major advantage of
   this test, particularly in infants. It has been used for the diagnosis
   of congenital adrenal hyperplasia (21-hydroxylase deficiency)
   but it is not specific.
● *24-h urinary steroid profile by GC-MS*
   The specific analysis of urinary steroid metabolites by gas
   chromatography–mass spectrometry (GC-MS) is the definitive
   method to delineate steroid enzymatic defects. The technique is
   available in a few specialized centres.

DYNAMIC TESTS

Stimulation Tests

   These are performed either to demonstrate adrenal insufficiency or to
delineate an enzyme deficiency by producing an increase in precursor
steroid production.

Short ACTH Stimulation (Synacthen Stimulation)

● Fasting not required
● Collect baseline blood for plasma cortisol ($t = 0$ min)
● Give Synacthen (tetracosactrin) 250 µg i.v. or i.m.
   Dose for infants 250 $\mu g/m^2$ or 36 µg/kg
● Collect blood at $t = 30, 60$ min.
   Interpretation: A normal response is a 2–3-fold increase
   in cortisol concentration. Saliva samples can also be used
   for cortisol measurement. There is a 7-fold increment in
   saliva cortisol concentration due to the greater proportion of
   free cortisol which is reflected by saliva measurement. If the
   response is subnormal, adrenal insufficiency is present. This is
   primary adrenal if ACTH levels are increased. The response
   may also be subnormal in secondary adrenal insufficiency
   (pituitary ACTH deficiency), particularly if long-standing.
   Other plasma steroids can be measured during this test if indicated,
e.g. 17-hydroxyprogesterone, androstenedione and testosterone in
suspected 21-hydroxylase deficiency; 11-deoxycortisol in suspected
11 β-hydroxylase deficiency.

Occasionally an i.v. infusion of ACTH over 4 or 6 hours is used as a stimulus. Synacthen 400 μg is infused i.v. Collect blood samples at 0, 4, and 6 hours.

Prolonged ACTH Stimulation

This test is indicated if the cortisol response to short ACTH stimulation is inadequate and secondary adrenal insufficiency is suspected.

- Fasting is not required
- Collect baseline blood sample for plasma cortisol ($t = 0$ min)
- Give Synacthen Depot (tetracosactrin acetate) 1 mg i.m. daily for 3 days. Mix well before injection.
- Collect blood for plasma cortisol 4–6 hours after the last Synacthen injection.

  Interpretation: Plasma cortisol increases at least 3-fold over basal concentrations in normals. There is also a response in secondary adrenal insufficiency. An absent cortisol response is definitive evidence of primary adrenal insufficiency.

If urinary steroid measurements are to be performed as an index of adrenal response, the following protocol should be used.

- Collect 2×24-h baseline urine samples for 17-OHCS, 17-OGS or urinary free cortisol and creatinine (days 1, 2)
- Give Synacthen Depot 1 mg i.m. daily for 3 days (days 3, 4, 5)
- Repeat 2×24-h urine collections starting on day 5 (days 5, 6).

  Interpretation: A normal response is a 2–3-fold increase in urinary steroid excretion by days 5 and 6.

- GC-MS profiles of the 24-h urine samples performed if an adrenal enzyme defect suspected.

Suppression Tests

These have been described in Chapter 2 in the section on ACTH secretion (pp. 16–17). They are:

Overnight dexamethasone suppression (for screening)
Low-dose dexamethasone suppression
High-dose dexamethasone suppression.

It is useful to have a sequence of steps for:
Confirmation of hypercortisolism
Investigation of the cause.

A suggested scheme for the investigation of Cushing's syndrome in childhood is presented in *Fig.* 5.4.

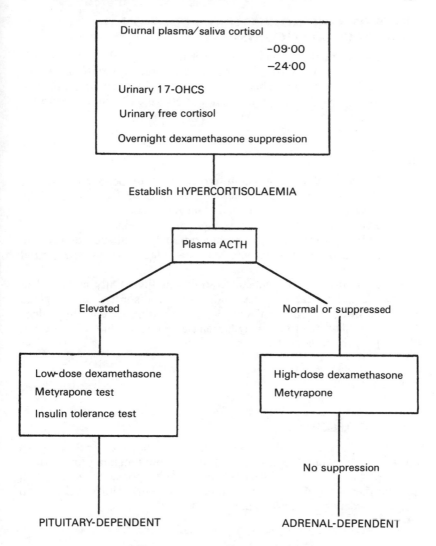

Fig. 5.4. Flow chart for investigation of Cushing's syndrome.

TESTS OF ADRENOCORTICAL FUNCTION (MINERALOCORTICOIDS)

Mineralocorticoid biosynthesis occurs in the zona glomerulosa via a series of enzymatic steps (*Fig.* 5.3) and is predominantly under the control of the renin–angiotensin system (*Fig.* 5.5). In children, tests of mineralocorticoid secretion are usually performed to investigate salt-losing states, and rarely for hypertension.

BASAL TESTS

- Plasma sodium, potassium, creatinine, bicarbonate and pH
- Plasma renin and aldosterone; in older children, this should be performed in the supine and erect positions
- 24-h urinary sodium, potassium and creatinine
- Other specific plasma mineralocorticoids, such as corticosterone and deoxycorticosterone, can be measured in specialized centres
- 24-h urinary mineralocorticoid metabolites. Only measured in specialized laboratories. Indicated for disorders affecting the pathway of mineralocorticoid biosynthesis, e.g. hypoaldosteronism due to 18-dehydrogenase deficiency and for suspected pseudohypoaldosteronism.

DYNAMIC TESTS

These are based on sodium balance studies. They require the services of a dietician experienced in designing and implementing low sodium diets, particularly in children. Usually the response to a restricted sodium diet is measured, for example in patients with CAH and no clinical evidence of salt losing.

Sodium Restriction

- Baseline
  - Plasma electrolytes
  - Plasma renin activity (PRA)
  - Plasma aldosterone
  - 24-h urine for electrolytes and creatinine (Day 1)
- Start low sodium diet—10–20 mmol/day (80–100 mmol/day potassium)

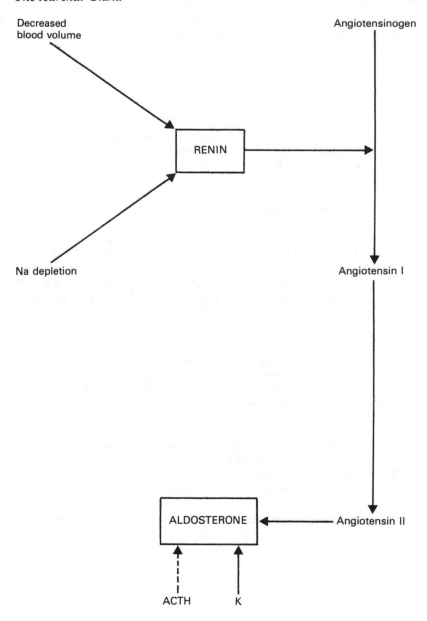

Fig. 5.5. Control of aldosterone secretion.

- Continue for 3 days (Days 2–4)
- Repeat 2 × 24-h urine collections for electrolytes, creatinine (Days 5, 6)
- Collect morning blood samples after patient in erect position for 1 hour for:
  Plasma electrolytes
  Plasma renin activity
  Plasma aldosterone (Days 5, 6)
  Interpretation: After 3 days sodium restriction, urinary sodium excretion usually falls below 10–20 mmol/day in normals. The plasma aldosterone and PRA increases at *least* three-fold.
  NB The following points are to be noted:
  It is very important to obtain sodium dietary intake 20 mmol/day or less
  Equilibrium with low sodium intake takes at least 3 days
  The rise in PRA with sodium restriction is only observed if the patient has been standing before the sample is collected
  For PRA, blood must be collected into chilled heparinized tubes, centrifuged at 4 °C and the plasma stored frozen until assay.
- If sodium is not conserved, fludrocortisone can be given 0·05 mg twice or three times daily. Baseline investigations should be repeated in 2 weeks to assess response to treatment.

Acute depletion of sodium by diuretic therapy or conversely, sodium loading tests using saline infusion, are not advisable in children.

Primary hyperaldosteronism (Conn's syndrome) is rare in children. If suspected the investigations required are:

- Plasma and urinary electrolytes (particularly potassium)
- Morning blood samples for PRA and aldosterone collected in the supine and erect positions
- Adrenal venography and selective bilateral venous sampling for plasma aldosterone measurements to localize an adrenal adenoma
- Other tests sometimes performed include [^{131}I]iodocholesterol and CT scanning.

ADRENAL MEDULLA

The adrenal medulla synthesizes catecholamines which can be measured directly in plasma or, more commonly, their metabolites are

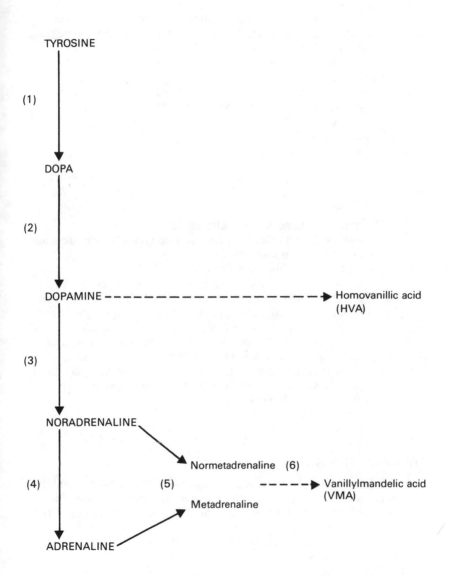

Fig. 5.6. Pathway of catecholamine synthesis and metabolism.

measured in urine. In children, investigation of the adrenal medulla is required for:
- Hypertension due to phaeochromocytoma
- Neuroblastoma

Fig. 5.6 illustrates the principal pathway of catecholamine synthesis and the metabolic products which are of relevance for diagnostic tests. Enzymes involved:
1. Tyrosine hydroxylase
2. Dopa decarboxylase
3. Dopamine β-hydroxylase
4. Phenylethanolamine-N-methyltransferase
5. Catechol-O-methyltransferase
6. Monoamine oxidase.

BASAL TESTS
- Plasma adrenaline and noradrenaline
- 24-h urinary total catecholamines (adrenaline and noradrenaline)
- 24-h urinary total metadrenaline
- 24-h urinary vanillylmandelic acid (VMA).

    Interpretation: Blood samples should be collected with the patient supine and resting after an overnight fast. Collect into chilled tubes and centrifuge at 4 °C to separate the plasma. Urine should be collected over 2×24-h consecutive periods into bottles containing acid. The patient should not be receiving any medication before or during these investigations. Foods such as bananas and icecream should be excluded. In children with phaeochromocytoma, the predominant catecholamine is usually noradrenaline.

DYNAMIC TESTS

Provocative tests, such as glucagon, histamine or tyramine stimulation are potentially dangerous and not indicated in children. Other investigations, particularly to delineate the site of a phaeochromocytoma (or a neuroblastoma) include:
- Plain abdominal radiograph and IVP
- CT scanning
- Ultrasound
- Selective venous sampling for catecholamine measurements
- Scintiscan using [^{131}I]metaiodobenzylguanidine.

CASE ILLUSTRATIONS

1. Pituitary-dependent Cushing's disease
2. Simple exogenous obesity
3. Addison's disease
4. Salt-losing congenital adrenal hyperplasia (male)
   21-Hydroxylase deficiency
5. Salt-losing congenital adrenal hyperplasia
   21-Hydroxylase deficiency
6. Late-onset congenital adrenal hyperplasia
7. Congenital adrenal hyperplasia
   11 β-Hydroxylase deficiency
8. Phaeochromocytoma

1. DIAGNOSIS: PITUITARY-DEPENDENT
CUSHING'S DISEASE

CASE HISTORY

A boy aged 12·7 years was referred for investigation of short stature and obesity. He was a full-term infant, birth weight 3240 g, who started to become obese at age 7 years. He previously was not small for his age but had stopped growing about 2 years before presentation. Headaches had developed recently. His parents were of average size.

His height was 130·4 cm ($-2·66$ s.d.) and weight 45·0 kg (75th centile). He had a round face, acne, truncal obesity and bruises on his limbs. Blood pressure was 130/80. Pubic hair was Tanner stage 4, but testes measured 2 ml in volume bilaterally. Bone age was 10·5 years. He had been previously investigated for suspected GH deficiency when a peak GH response of 3·7 mU/l was obtained with hypoglycaemia of 1·5 mmol/l.

INITIAL INVESTIGATIONS AND RESULTS

- Hb 15·9 g/dl
  RBC 5·75 × 10^{12}/l
  PCV 45·4
- Plasma

Urea	5·5 mmol/l
Na	135 mmol/l
K	3·5 mmol/l
- Radiograph skull *normal*
- Plasma cortisol
  09:00—940 nmol/l
  24:00—720 nmol/l

FURTHER INVESTIGATIONS

- Low-dose dexamethasone suppression
- High-dose dexamethasone suppression
- Metyrapone test
- Bilateral adrenal venogram.

RESULTS

Test	Plasma		Urine	
	Cortisol nmol/l	ACTH ng/l	Cortisol derivatives mmol/mol creat.	Cortisol precursors mmol/mol creat.
Low-dose Dex.				
Pre-	720	150	9·1	0·7
Post-	195	34	0·8	0·4
High-dose Dex.				
Post-	55	< 6·0	0·2	0·1
Metyrapone				
Pre-	—	—	6·2	0·3
Post-	—	—	4·8	18·2
		(N<10–80)	(N 1·6–4·4)	(N 0·2–0·6)

Bilateral adrenal venogram
There was no evidence of an adrenal mass. Plasma cortisol was determined in selective blood samples obtained from the following sites:

Right adrenal vein	2000 nmol/l
Right renal vein	480 nmol/l
Left adrenal vein	2000 nmol/l
Left renal vein	1080 nmol/l
IVC above adrenals	565 nmol/l
IVC below adrenals	430 nmol/l

COMMENT

The combination of obesity and short stature, hypertension, elevated plasma cortisol levels at midnight and increased urinary excretion of cortisol metabolites indicated Cushing's *syndrome*. The cause was established using additional dynamic tests of adrenal function. Adrenal suppression was readily achieved with low-dose dexamethasone. Plasma ACTH levels were elevated and also suppressed readily. The absence of an adrenal mass on venography, and no unilateral high gradient in plasma cortisol concentrations at selective venous sites, suggested pituitary-dependent bilateral adrenal hyperplasia (Cushing's *disease*) as the cause.

Bilateral adrenalectomy was performed. Hyperplastic adrenals were confirmed histologically. He was given maintenance hydrocortisone and 9 α-fludrocortisone therapy long-term. Puberty developed spontaneously; at 18·0 years his final height is 165·0 cm (10th centile). To date, there has been no evidence for the development of a pituitary adenoma and hyperpigmentation (Nelson's syndrome). Nowadays the preferred treatment of choice in Cushing's disease is trans-sphenoidal microadenomectomy.

The details of this case were kindly provided by Dr D. C. L. Savage, Paediatric Endocrinologist, Bristol.

2. DIAGNOSIS: SIMPLE EXOGENOUS OBESITY

CASE HISTORY

A boy was referred at age 12·7 years for simple obesity. His birth weight was 3580 g. He had generalized obesity and a few red striae over the abdomen and thighs. He was not hirsute. Blood pressure when first recorded was 180/100 but subsequent readings were 130/70. His height was 141·5 cm (− 1·18 s.d.) and weight 65·7 kg (> 97th centile). Bone age was 10·4 years. Radiographs of the skull and spine were normal.

INVESTIGATIONS AND RESULTS

- Plasma cortisol
      08:00—1200 nmol/l
      24:00— 300 nmol/l
- 24-h urinary-free cortisol 230 nmol/l
- Overnight dexamethasone suppression
      1 mg dexamethasone orally at 24:00
   Plasma cortisol
      24:00—370 nmol/l
      08:00— 30 nmol/l

COMMENT

As a general rule, simple obesity is associated with normal or tall stature. In contrast, endocrine-related obesity is usually accompanied by short stature. Examples include hypothyroidism, GH deficiency, pseudohypoparathyroidism and Cushing's syndrome. The latter diagnosis was considered in this boy because he was short and possibly hypertensive. Previous growth measurements, however, showed that his height and weight were on the 10th and 50th centiles, respectively, at age 6 years. There was a normal diurnal rhythm in plasma cortisol levels which suppressed normally following overnight dexamethasone. The 24-h urinary free cortisol concentration was not elevated. A calorie-reducing diet was started.

3. DIAGNOSIS: ADDISON'S DISEASE

CASE HISTORY

A boy aged 7 years was investigated for tiredness and lethargy, recurrent abdominal pain, weight loss and constipation. These symptoms had been present for at least a year; his previous health was normal. He was noted to be generally pigmented. Blood pressure was 110/80 supine, and 90/70 in the erect position. Radiograph of the skull was normal.

INVESTIGATIONS AND RESULTS

- Hb 9·8 g/dl
  PCV 38·2
  Blood film—normochromia
- Plasma
  - Urea   8·0   mmol/l
  - Ca   2·40 mmol/l
- Serum
  - Na   128 mmol/l
  - K   6·0   mmol/l
  - Cl   92 mmol/l
- Plasma glucose (fasting) 2·2 mmol/l
- Plasma ACTH 420 ng/l (*normal* 10–80 ng/l)
- Serum
  - TSH   3·8 mU/l
  - T_4 118 nmol/l
- Short ACTH stimulation
  Synacthen 250 μg i.m.
  Plasma cortisol
  - 0 min—< 28 nmol/l
  - 60 min—< 28 nmol/l
- Prolonged ACTH stimulation
  Synacthen Depot 1 mg i.m. daily for 3 days
  Plasma cortisol
  - Basal—< 28 nmol/l
  - Post-ACTH—< 28 nmol/l
- Auto-antibodies
  - Adrenal microsomal   *positive* 1/64
  - Thyroid microsomal   *positive* 1/64
  - Parietal cell   *negative*
  - Islet cell   *negative*
  - Ovarian   *negative*

COMMENT

Addison's disease is very uncommon in children. This boy's symptoms were rather non-specific; however the pigmentation was quite striking, particularly affecting the areola and scrotal skin. He had no symptoms of hypoglycaemia, but fasting plasma glucose was low. There was a normochromic anaemia, hyponatraemia and hyperkalaemia. Plasma calcium was normal. The diagnosis of primary adrenal failure was confirmed by a marked increase in plasma ACTH and the absent plasma cortisol response to exogenous ACTH (short- and long-term). The presence of adrenal antibodies indicated auto-immune Addison's disease. Although he is euthyroid the boy is at risk of developing associated hypothyroidism (Schmidt's syndrome) due to the presence of thyroid auto-antibodies. He was treated with hydrocortisone (10 mg morning, 5 mg evening) and 9 α-fludrocortisone daily.

4. DIAGNOSIS: SALT-LOSING CONGENITAL ADRENAL HYPERPLASIA (MALE) 21-HYDROXYLASE DEFICIENCY

CASE HISTORY

A male infant, birth weight 3310 g, was born at term following a normal pregnancy. An emergency caesarian section was performed because of fetal distress. He was breast fed and the early neonatal period was uneventful. Poor weight gain was noted in hospital. This persisted despite supplementation with bottle milk feeds. At age 4 weeks, his weight had decreased to 2920 g. He was the first born to unrelated parents. There was no relevant family history. He was clinically dehydrated and wasted. The external genitalia were normal for a male infant.

INVESTIGATIONS AND RESULTS

- Plasma

Urea	6·5 mmol/l
Na	106 mmol/l
K	7·5 mmol/l
Glucose	5·2 mmol/l

- Plasma

17OH-Progesterone	700 nmol/l
Testosterone	26 nmol/l

- Plasma renin activity   58 pmol/h per ml

COMMENT

The clinical problem was failure to gain weight despite adequate feeds, dehydration and severe hyponatraemia and hyperkalaemia. He had also vomited twice. There were no clinical signs of pyloric stenosis and the electrolyte pattern was not typical for that disorder. A marked increase in plasma 17OH-progesterone confirmed the diagnosis. The plasma testosterone concentration was *above* the upper limit of the normal adult male range. Too frequently in the past, the diagnosis of salt-losing congenital adrenal hyperplasia in a male infant has been missed. The infant was rehydrated with intravenous normal saline; replacement therapy with hydrocortisone and 9 α-fludrocortisone was started. Six weeks later plasma 17OH-progesterone and testosterone concentrations were 13 nmol/l and 0·6 nmol/l, respectively.

5. DIAGNOSIS: SALT-LOSING CONGENITAL ADRENAL HYPERPLASIA 21-HYDROXYLASE DEFICIENCY

CASE HISTORY

A full-term infant, birth weight 2720 g, was born at home following a normal pregnancy. The external genitalia were noted to be abnormal but the mother was told that the infant was 'probably' a boy. Referred for further investigation at age 2 weeks. The phallus was small and bound down by a chordee. Pigmented, rugose labioscrotal folds encircled the phallus; no gonads were palpable. There was a single opening on the perineum. The infant was clinically dehydrated.

INVESTIGATIONS AND RESULTS

- Plasma

Urea	7·7 mmol/l
Na	127 mmol/l
K	7·1 mmol/l
Glucose	4·9 mmol/l

- Peripheral karyotype 46 XX
- Plasma

17OH-Progesterone	670 nmol/l
Testosterone	8 nmol/l

- Plasma renin activity 64 pmol/h per ml (N < 30 for age)

COMMENT

The diagnosis in an infant with ambiguous genitalia and salt-wasting is most likely congenital adrenal hyperplasia due to 21-hydroxylase deficiency. A much rarer possibility is 3βol-hydroxysteroid dehydrogenase deficiency. The diagnosis was confirmed by a female karyotype and a markedly elevated plasma 17OH-progesterone concentration (normal < 15 nmol/l). Measurement of this steroid in plasma is a rapid and reliable diagnostic test for 21-hydroxylase deficiency. Occasional spurious elevations are observed in very sick infants (particularly preterm) who are ill due to non-adrenal causes. Most laboratories that assay 17OH-progesterone can now provide a result within 24 h of blood sample collection. Plasma renin activity was also elevated as a result of hyponatraemia and dehydration. The infant was rehydrated with intravenous saline and replacement therapy started with hydrocortisone and 9α-fludrocortisone. Within 3 weeks, plasma 17OH-progesterone and testosterone concentrations had decreased to 60 nmol/l and 1·5 nmol/l respectively. Clitoral recession and a vaginoplasty were performed at age 6 months.

6. DIAGNOSIS: LATE-ONSET CONGENITAL ADRENAL HYPERPLASIA

CASE HISTORY

A female developed pubic hair at age 4 years. She also started treatment with sodium valproate (an anticonvulsant) at this time because of recurrent febrile convulsions. This produced downy hair growth on limbs which disappeared when valproate therapy was discontinued. Pubic hair growth continued. When referred at age 7·4 years, height was 124·1 cm (+ 0·39 s.d.). Pubic hair and breast development were Tanner stages 2 and 1, respectively. There was minimal clitoromegaly, but no labial fusion. Blood pressure was normal. Bone age 9·8 years. Plasma urea and electrolytes were normal.

INVESTIGATIONS

- Short ACTH stimulation test
  Synacthen 250 µg i.m.
- Prolonged ACTH stimulation test
  Synacthen Depot 1 mg daily for 3 days
- Low-dose dexamethasone suppression test
  0·5 mg every 6 hours for 2 days
- Short ACTH stimulation test (parents and siblings)
- Family HLA typing.

COMMENT

The possible causes of early pubic hair growth include premature adrenarche, androgen-secreting adrenal tumour and late-onset congenital adrenal hyperplasia. Premature adrenarche was unlikely in the presence of clitoromegaly, but compatible with an advanced bone age. Basal plasma and saliva 17OH-progesterone levels were elevated, and the plasma testosterone concentration was increased for a prepubertal female. Plasma dehydroepiandrosterone and its sulphate, which are usually elevated in premature adrenarche, were not determined. Short

RESULTS

Time	Plasma				Saliva	
	Cortisol	17-OHP	Andro-stenedione	Testos-terone	Cortisol	17-OHP
min	nmol/l	nmol/l	nmol/l	nmol/l	nmol/l	nmol/l
Short ACTH						
0	267	64	4·6	1·4	4·7	1570
30	397	84	5·0	1·6	50	1500
60	485	87	5·8	2·0	56	2770
120	437	61	5·2	1·5	50	1930
Prolonged ACTH						
Post-ACTH	1200	54	9·0	2·3	110	1440
Dexamethasone suppression						
Post-dex	45	2	4·4	0·9	1·5	< 150

● Short ACTH stimulation test (parents and siblings)
  Synacthen 250 µg i.m. given to:
    Father
    Mother (during follicular phase of cycle)
    Sister (aged 5·5 years)

Plasma	Time min	Father	Mother	Sister (5·5 years)	Sister (3·0 years)
Cortisol,	0	172	159	131	—
nmol/l	60	802	488	625	—
17-OHP	0	2·5	2·1	2·3	0·9
nmol/l	60	22·2	11·6	19·9	—
Androstenedione,	0	3·4	2·4	1·6	—
nmol/l	60	7·3	5·3	2·3	—
Testosterone,	0	8·0	1·2	0·5	0·4
nmol/l	60	11·0	1·5	0·9	—
Saliva	Time min				
Cortisol,	0	5·5	3·2	4·7	—
nmol/l	60	37·0	42·0	29·1	—
17-OHP,	0	< 150	< 150	< 150	< 150
pmol/l	60	833	387	833	—

Another sister, aged 3·0 years, had basal samples collected only.

● Family HLA Typing

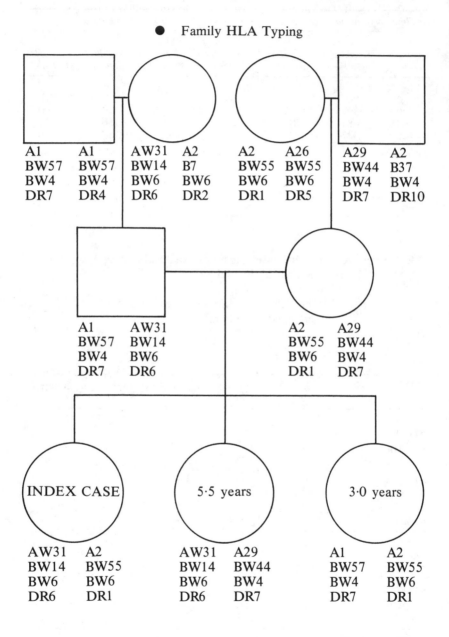

and longer-term ACTH stimulation caused an increase in steroid precursors and androgens; the normal plasma and saliva cortisol response indicate that 21-hydroxylase deficiency is partial. Low-dose dexamethasone produced complete suppression of steroid concentrations in plasma and saliva, thus excluding an adrenal tumour.

Family studies were performed in order to detect heterozygotes for 21-hydroxylase deficiency. The parents were obligate heterozygotes. Both parents and the sister (age 5·5 years) showed a 17OH-progesterone response within the range obtained in heterozygotes for the late-onset variant of this disorder. Genetic linkage between the HLA complex and the alleles for 21-hydroxylase deficiency is well established. Thus the index case, her two sisters, parents, and both sets of grandparents were HLA genotyped. Antigens of the HLA-A, -B, -C, -DR loci were determined using standard reference methods. Survey of the haplotypes shows that both sisters are heterozygotes. For example, the older sibling (5·5 years) shares antigens AW31, BW14, BW6, DR6 with the index case; these in turn have been inherited from the father and paternal grandmother.

cDNA probes are now available to study the cytochrome P450 21-hydroxylase gene in congenital adrenal hyperplasia. Digestion of genomic DNA from family members using a range of restriction enzymes has shown that one third to one half of patients with the classical form of 21-hydroxylase deficiency have a gene deletion. This type of analysis is also useful for detecting heterozygotes and for early prenatal diagnosis by using material from a chorionic villus biopsy as the source of DNA.

The index case was started on cortisone acetate, 2·5 mg twice daily. Concentrations of plasma 17OH-progesterone and testosterone decreased to 4·0 and 0·8 nmol/l, respectively.

7. DIAGNOSIS: CONGENITAL ADRENAL HYPERPLASIA 11β-HYDROXYLASE DEFICIENCY

CASE HISTORY

A full-term infant, birth weight 2450 g, first born to unrelated Indian parents was noted to have ambiguous genitalia. The pregnancy was normal and there was no relevant family history. There was a 2 cm long phallus with a dimple on the ventral surface of the glans. Pigmented, slightly rugose labioscrotal folds were present; no gonads were palpable. There was a single perineal opening through which the infant voided urine. The remainder of the examination, including blood pressure, was normal.

INVESTIGATIONS AND RESULTS
- Serial serum electrolytes *normal*
- Peripheral karyotype 46 XX
- Perineal sinogram: a common urogenital sinus was demonstrated; a long and distensible vagina/cervix/uterus was outlined
- Plasma steroids

17OH-Progesterone	14 nmol/l
Cortisol	848 nmol/l
Testosterone	7·7 nmol/l
11-Deoxycortisol	> 2000 nmol/l

- 24-h urinary steroids (measured by gas chromatography)

Tetrahydro-11-deoxycortisol	380 μg/day (N < 50)
6 α-hydroxytetrahydro-11-deoxycortisol	700 μg/day (N < 50)
Pregnanetriol	0·08 μg/day (*normal*)

COMMENT

A preliminary report on the karyotype was available within 48 h of lymphocyte culture. In the absence of a maternal source of androgens, virilization in a 46 XX infant is due to congenital adrenal hyperplasia. A normal plasma 17OH-progesterone concentration (< 15 nmol/l) excluded 21-hydroxylase deficiency. The diagnosis was clinched by markedly elevated concentrations of 11-deoxycortisol in plasma and its metabolites in urine. Virilization resulted from the increased secretion of testosterone. Salt loss did not occur because of increased production of mineralocorticoids such as deoxycorticosterone. This did not cause hypertension, but would have done so later had the infant not been treated. The radiographic demonstration of normal female internal genitalia was convincing evidence for these particular parents that the infant should be reared as female. Treatment was started with a daily replacement dose of hydrocortisone. Clitoral recession and vaginoplasty were performed at age 7 months.

The enzyme deficiency is an autosomal recessive disorder. The parents did not wish prenatal diagnosis during a subsequent pregnancy. An infant with ambiguous genitalia was born at term. A 46 XX karyotype, elevated plasma 11-deoxycortisol, testosterone but normal 17OH-progesterone, and increased urinary excretion of tetrahydro-11-deoxycortisol confirmed the diagnosis of 11β-hydroxylase deficiency.

8. DIAGNOSIS: PHAEOCHROMOCYTOMA

CASE HISTORY

A boy aged 10 years was referred because of excessive perspiration. This had been present for 6 months and was worse at night. There was no weight loss; he had some nocturia. Apart from some recent headaches, his general health was normal.

The only abnormality found on examination was a blood pressure of 170/120 mmHg.

INVESTIGATIONS AND RESULTS

> Chest radiograph—*normal*
> Electrocardiograph—*normal*
> Intravenous pyelography: soft tissue mass at upper pole of right kidney
> ● Serum T_4 102 nmol/l
> Urinary VMA 51 μmol/day (N 0–35)
> VMA/creatinine ratio 17·3 (*increased*)
> Urinary metadrenaline 42·0 μmol/day (N 0–6·5)
> Serum calcitonin 0·15 μg/l (N < 0·08)
> CT scan: large mass superior to right kidney.

COMMENT

Hypertension in childhood requires detailed investigation. Symptoms and signs of phaeochromocytoma in childhood are usually persistent. This was the likeliest diagnosis in a hypertensive child with excessive perspiration. The anatomical location was confirmed by radiography and CT scanning. Increased catecholamine production was confirmed. He was started on phenoxybenzamine and propanolol to produce full α- and β-blockade before general anaesthesia. After 2–3 weeks, his blood pressure was 100/80 in the erect and 70/40 mmHg in the supine positions, respectively. At operation the right adrenal gland was replaced by a large lobulated firm tumour which was well encapsulated. This was excised. The left adrenal gland was normal; no other masses were seen after extensive inspection of para-aortic and paracaval regions and the pelvis. Histology showed the features of a phaeochromocytoma. He made an uneventful recovery and remains well and normotensive. Urinary VMA and metadrenaline concentrations are normal. Serum calcitonin was slightly increased pre-operatively, but subsequent measurements have been normal. There is no evidence of associated thyroid medullary carcinoma.

The details of this case were kindly provided by Dr J. A. Dodge, Reader in Child Health, Cardiff.

CHAPTER 6

The Gonads

The clinical evaluation of gonadal function is essential before undertaking specific tests of testicular or gonadal function. The reader must be familiar with the signs of pubertal development in both sexes, particularly as documented in detail by Tanner.[1]

TESTIS

Testicular function is under the control of GnRH (LHRH) via pituitary LH and FSH secretion.

Testosterone biosynthesis by the Leydig cells of the testis proceeds via a sequence of enzymatic steps under the control of LH secretion. The pathways of testicular steroid biosynthesis are shown in *Fig.* 6.1. There is a negative feedback of testosterone on LH secretion both directly at the pituitary and indirectly at the hypothalamic level. The feedback relationship is developed in early infancy.

BASAL INVESTIGATIONS

- Plasma testosterone
- Plasma androstenedione
- Plasma dihydrotestosterone
- Plasma oestradiol
- Serum LH and FSH.

   Interpretation: In primary testicular failure, basal gonado-trophins may be elevated. Normally, prepubertal boys have low plasma testosterone concentrations although there is a surge in levels from birth to 3 months of age. There is a gradual increase in plasma testosterone concentrations at the time of puberty, but single random determinations are of little value to document the onset of puberty.

DYNAMIC TESTS

LHRH Stimulation

(*See* Chapter 2, p. 17).

   Interpretation: The peak LH and FSH responses increase with

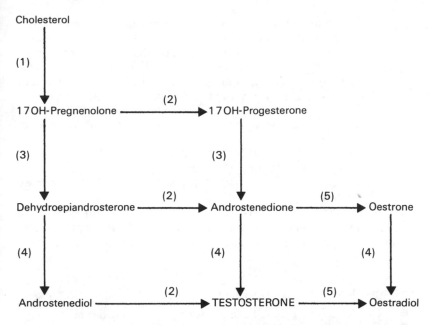

Fig. 6.1. Pathway of testosterone biosynthesis. Enzymes: (1) desmolase; (2) 3β-hydroxysteroid dehydrogenase; (3) 17, 20-desmolase; (4) 17β-hydroxysteroid dehydrogenase; (5) aromatase.

the onset of puberty. An absent response suggests hypogonadotrophic hypogonadism, but the results are not always clearly distinguished from those obtained in a normal boy with delayed puberty. An exaggerated LH/FSH response in the presence of low plasma testosterone concentrations indicates primary testicular failure. If facilities are available, profiles of pulsatile LH and FSH secretion (particularly nocturnal) provide added information on the progression of puberty.

HCG Stimulation

- Collect baseline blood sample for plasma testosterone (also androstenedione, and dihydrotestosterone if steroid biosynthetic defect suspected) (Day 1)
- Give HCG (Pregnyl) 2000 units i.m. daily for 3 days (Day 1, 2, 3)
- Repeat blood sample 24 h after last injection (Day 4).
    Interpretation: Plasma testosterone increases at least two–

three-fold following HCG stimulation in prepubertal boys. The response is more marked in male infants age 0–6 months and during early to mid-puberty. An absent response with an exaggerated LH/FSH response to LHRH stimulation indicates primary gonadal failure or anorchia. If there is a defect in testosterone biosynthesis, there will be an increase in precursor steroid secretion following HCG stimulation. Results can be expressed as a ratio of steroid precursor to product concentration, e.g.:

- Increased androstenedione: testosterone ratio—17β-hydroxysteroid dehydrogenase deficiency.
- Increased testosterone: dihydrotestosterone ratio—5α-reductase deficiency.

Baseline and post-HCG 24-h urine samples for measurement of the specific urinary metabolites of these steroids by GC-MS is particularly useful to delineate a defect in androgen biosynthesis or metabolism.

Prolonged HCG Stimulation Test

- Collect baseline blood sample for plasma testosterone
- Give 2000 units HCG i.m. twice weekly for *3 weeks*
- Repeat blood sample 24 h after last injection.
  Interpretation: Occasionally there will be a testosterone response during the prolonged test when the response was absent in the short HCG stimulation test. A completely absent response confirms functional primary hypogonadism. The test is also useful in the investigation of boys with bilateral cryptorchidism.

Other Tests of Testicular Function

- Karyotype—blood
             —skin fibroblasts
  e.g. 47 XXY (Klinefelter),
        47 XY/XXY mosaicism
- Seminal analysis (appropriate only in postpuberty)
- Testicular biopsy
- DNA analysis using Y-specific cDNA probes, particularly for the testis-determining gene (TDF)
- Androgen receptors in genital skin fibroblasts.

Note: These last 2 investigations are available only in specialized centres; they have a special role in the investigation of the 46XX male and the 46XY female with absent or incomplete virilization.

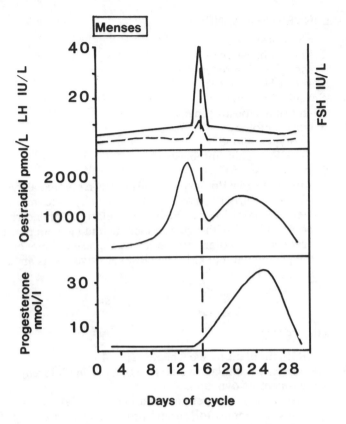

Fig. 6.2. Hormone profiles during normal adult menstrual cycle. In top profile (—) luteinizing hormone, (----) follicle-stimulating hormone.

OVARY

Unlike the testis, ovarian activity is minimal during childhood. Oestradiol, progesterone and androstenedione are the principal steroids secreted by the ovary under pituitary LH/FSH control. Ovarian steroids are secreted in a cyclical fashion at the time of full maturation of the hypothalamo–pituitary–ovarian axis soon after menarche. The gonado-trophin and steroid profiles typical in the adult menstrual cycle are shown in *Fig.* 6.2.

BASAL INVESTIGATIONS

- Plasma oestradiol
- Plasma progesterone
- Plasma 17 OH-progesterone
- Serum LH and FSH
- Serum prolactin
- 24-h urinary oestrogens
- Vaginal cytology
- Karyotype—blood
　　　　　　—skin fibroblasts
- Pelvic ultrasound.

　　　Interpretation: Primary gonadal failure (e.g. gonadal dysgenesis 45 XO, Turner's syndrome) is usually accompanied by elevated basal LH and FSH (particularly). Amenorrhoea can be associated with hyperprolactinaemia (uncommon in children). Do not forget *pregnancy* as a cause of amenorrhoea in the postmenarchal girl. The most sensitive test is an assay for serum β-HCG.

DYNAMIC TESTS

- LHRH stimulation (*see* Chapter 2, p. 17)
- Clomiphene stimulation (rarely indicated in children)
- Assessment of ovulation
　　　　Basal body temperature chart (unreliable)
　　　　Blood samples for plasma progesterone on days 3–5, and 21–23 of the menstrual cycle
　　　　Daily saliva sample collection throughout menstrual cycle for progesterone profile
　　　　Ovarian ultrasound.

　　　Interpretation: Assessment of ovulation is rarely indicated in children. Certain conditions such as diabetes mellitus and congenital adrenal hyperplasia if poorly controlled in post-menarche, can cause anovulation.

DISORDERS OF SEXUAL DIFFERENTIATION

　It is convenient to list the investigations appropriate for these disorders in this Chapter, even though the commonest cause of ambiguous genitalia is congenital adrenal hyperplasia (CAH)—an adrenal disorder (*see Fig.* 6.3).

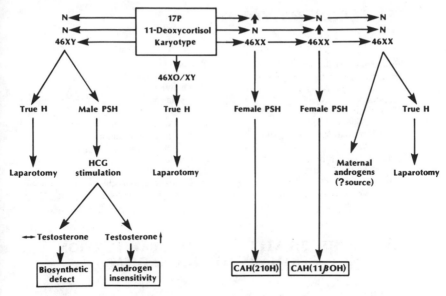

Fig. 6.3. Flow diagram for investigation of ambiguous genitalia.

AMBIGUOUS GENITALIA

- Karyotype in peripheral blood. A buccal smear for Barr bodies *is not reliable*
- Plasma 17 OH-progesterone
- Plasma 11-deoxycortisol
- Plasma electrolytes, plasma renin activity
- Random urine for 11-oxygenation index, electrolytes
- 24-h urine for 17-OS, pregnanetriol, tetrahydro-11-deoxycortisol
- HCG stimulation (if karyotype is 46 XY)

  Interpretation: Commonest cause of ambiguous genitalia of the newborn is CAH; most frequent enzyme deficiency causing CAH is 21-hydroxylase deficiency.

  An elevated plasma 17 OH progesterone concentration in a 46 XX infant is due to 21-hydroxylase deficiency.

  A flow diagram of investigations is shown in *Fig.* 6.3.

  NB Investigations to be performed *promptly* so that an early decision on the sex of rearing can be taken.

Reference

Tanner J. M. (1962) *Growth at Adolescence,* 2nd edn. Oxford: Blackwell Scientific.

CASE ILLUSTRATIONS

1. Bilateral testicular torsion
   Primary hypogonadism
2. Bilateral cryptorchidism
3. Isolated micropenis
4. Isolated micropenis
5. Pubertal gynaecomastia
6. Complete androgen insensitivity
   syndrome
   Androgen-receptor negative
7. Partial androgen insensitivity
   syndrome
   Androgen-receptor positive
8. Ambiguous genitalia
   Mixed gonadal dysgenesis
9. Delayed puberty (female)
   Radiation-induced primary ovarian
   failure
10. Acute myeloid leukaemia
    Secondary lymphoma
    Radiation-induced primary ovarian
    failure
11. Premature thelarche
12. Premature thelarche
13. Idiopathic hirsutism

1. DIAGNOSIS: BILATERAL TESTICULAR TORSION
PRIMARY HYPOGONADISM

CASE HISTORY

A male infant was noted to have bilateral torsion of the testes soon after birth. The testes subsequently atrophied. When referred at age 7 years, there was a small gonad (< 0.5 cm length) palpable in the right hemiscrotum only. The penis was normal.

INVESTIGATIONS AND RESULTS

- Basal
  - Serum LH 4·8 U/l
  - FSH > 40 U/l
  - Plasma testosterone 0·8 nmol/l
- LHRH stimulation (100 μg i.v.)
  - Peak LH 36·7 U/l
  - Peak FSH > 40 U/l
- HCG stimulation (2000 units i.m. daily for 3 days)
  - Plasma testosterone
    - Pre-HCG 0·8 nmol/l
    - Post-HCG 0·9 nmol/l

COMMENT

This boy has primary hypogonadism. He will require androgen replacement to induce signs of puberty and testicular prostheses inserted. He will be infertile.

2. DIAGNOSIS: BILATERAL CRYPTORCHIDISM

CASE HISTORY

Bilateral exploration of the groins was performed on a 6-year-old boy with undescended testes. No testes or vasa deferentia were identified. The penis and scrotum were normal for a prepubertal boy.

INVESTIGATIONS

- Peripheral karyotype 46 XY
- LHRH stimulation
  100 μg i.v.
- Prolonged HCG stimulation
  2000 units i.m. twice weekly for 3 weeks.

RESULTS

Time min	LH U/l	FSH U/l	Test nmol/l
LHRH			
0	1·1	0·8	0·4
30	5·0	5·3	—
60	3·5	5·7	—
120	2·0	4·6	0·3
HCG			
Pre-			0·3
Post-			8·7

COMMENT

No testicular tissue was identified to resite in the scrotum. There is evidence of intra-abdominal tissue based on a normal prepubertal gonadotrophin response to LHRH and an increase in plasma testosterone following prolonged HCG stimulation. Adequate Leydig cell function in early fetal life is implicit on evidence of normal development of the external genitalia. It is possible that secondary sexual characteristics will develop spontaneously with endogenous testosterone production at the time of puberty. He will be infertile and will require insertion of testicular prostheses at the appropriate time. Whether intra-abdominal testicular tissue should be excised after puberty is debatable.

3. DIAGNOSIS: ISOLATED MICROPENIS

CASE HISTORY

Referred at age 13·0 years because of small genitalia. He had a right orchidopexy one year previously for an undescended testis. His growth was normal. There was no evidence of anosmia. He was prepubertal. The stretched penile length was 1·5 cm (< 2·5 s.d.). There was a flat scrotum containing a right testis 2 ml in volume. The left testis was retractile.

INVESTIGATIONS

- Peripheral karyotype
- LHRH stimulation test
    100 μg i.v.
- Short HCG stimulation test
    2000 units i.m. daily for 3 days
- Scrotal skin punch biopsy for
    Androgen receptor concentration (B_{max})
    Binding affinity (K_d)

RESULTS

- Karyotype 46 XY
- LHRH stimulation

Time min	LH U/l	FSH U/l	Testosterone nmol/l
0	1·3	0·8	1·0
30	3·3	3·3	—
60	2·4	3·2	—
120	1·4	2·7	0·5

- HCG stimulation
    Plasma testosterone
    Pre-HCG 0·7 nmol/l
    Post-HCG 7·2 nmol/l
- Scrotal genital skin fibroblasts
    Androgen receptor concentration (B_{max})
    998×10^{-18} mol/μg DNA (N 775 ± 185, mean ± s.d.)
    Binding affinity (K_d)
    $0·35 \times 10^{-10}$M (N 0·88 ± 0·35)

Note: There was a two-fold augmentation in androgen receptor binding activity when the cells were pre-incubated with androgens before assay.

COMMENT

There was no ambiguity of the external genitalia. The gonadotrophin response to LHRH stimulation was prepubertal and normal. Following short-term HCG stimulation, there was a satisfactory increase in plasma testosterone concentration thus excluding a defect in testosterone biosynthesis. Finally analysis of androgen receptor binding in scrotal skin fibroblasts showed there was no defect in peripheral action of androgens. The increase in binding activity demonstrated *in vitro* with androgen pre-incubation before assay suggested there should be a response *in vivo* to exogenous androgens. Treatment was started with Sustanon 50 mg i.m. each month. Within 6 months, penile size had increased to 6·0 cm stretched length.

4. DIAGNOSIS: ISOLATED MICROPENIS

CASE HISTORY

Referred at age 9·8 years because of concern with size of penis. Previous health normal. Stretched penile length 2·5 cm. Testes descended, measuring < 1·0 ml in volume bilaterally.

INVESTIGATIONS AND RESULTS

- Peripheral karyotype 46 XY
- LHRH stimulation (100 μg i.v.)
  - Peak LH   1·6 U/l
  - Peak FSH   4·5 U/l
- Short HCG stimulation (2000 units i.m. daily for 3 days)
  - Testosterone
    - Pre-HCG   0·9 nmol/l
    - Post-HCG   1·4 nmol/l
- Prolonged HCG stimulation (2000 units i.m. twice weekly for 3 weeks)
  - Testosterone
    - Pre-HCG   0·7 nmol/l
    - Post-HCG   10·0 nmol/l
- Androgen receptors in genital skin fibroblasts (punch biopsy)
  - Concentration (B_{max}) 791×10^{-18} mol/μg DNA (*normal*)
  - Binding affinity (K_d) $0·77 \times 10^{-10}$M (*normal*)

COMMENT

No abnormality has been found to account for the micropenis. There is a normal prepubertal gonadotrophin response to LHRH stimulation. The initial Leydig cell response to HCG stimulation was suboptimal, but with prolonged HCG stimulation there was an adequate increase in plasma testosterone. A scrotal skin bopsy (2 mm punch) was obtained under local anaesthetic and fibroblasts cultured. The concentration of androgen receptors and their affinity for radiolabelled DHT was normal. Consequently the stimulus for, the production of, and the intracellular action of androgens were all normal. The boy requires observation during puberty; he may require additional exogenous androgens to promote penile growth.

5. DIAGNOSIS: PUBERTAL GYNAECOMASTIA

CASE HISTORY

A boy aged 13·9 years was referred because of breast development. He was very embarrassed about this and had stopped swimming and playing sports in school. He was receiving no medication. There was bilateral gynaecomastia (5 cm diameter breast tissue) which was tender; there was no galactorrhoea. Pubic hair was Tanner stage 3; testes measured 15 ml in volume bilaterally. He was very thin (triceps and subscapular skinfolds < 3rd centile). Bone age was 14·0 years.

INVESTIGATIONS AND RESULTS

- Peripheral karyotype 46 XY
- Serum prolactin 80 mU/l
- Serum
    - LH   1·2 U/l
    - FSH   0·9 U/l
- Plasma
    - Testosterone 23 nmol/l
    - Oestradiol 174 pmol/l

COMMENT

Klinefelter's syndrome as the cause for gynaecomastia was excluded by a normal male karyotype. A normal serum prolactin and absence of galactorrhoea ruled out hyperprolactinaemia. Puberty was also advanced, he was growing rapidly and his plasma testosterone concentration was within the adult male range. This is characteristic of pubertal gynaecomastia which occurs in about 70 per cent of boys. Breast development was very evident because he was so thin. With the assistance of an Adolescent Child Psychiatrist it was possible to dissuade the boy from seeking bilateral mastectomy to solve the problem. He was able to adjust satisfactorily with the knowledge that the gynaecomastia would resolve spontaneously. Thus by age 16 years he was discharged from the clinic having completed puberty normally. There was no residual gynaecomastia.

6. DIAGNOSIS: COMPLETE ANDROGEN INSENSITIVITY SYNDROME ANDROGEN-RECEPTOR NEGATIVE

CASE HISTORY

A female infant presented at 10 days of age with bilateral swellings in the groins. These were more prominent when she cried. The external genitalia were normal for a female. She had 3 older sisters aged 2, 4 and 7 years. The 7-year-old sister had had bilateral inguinal herniae repaired at age 18 months.

INVESTIGATIONS AND RESULTS

- Peripheral karyotype
  Index case 46 XY
  Siblings
     7 years 46 XY
     4 years 46 XX
     2 years 46 XX
- Plasma testosterone 3·9 nmol/l
- Androgen receptors: No detectable specific androgen-receptor binding in labial skin fibroblasts from the index case and her 7-year-old sibling.

COMMENT

Bilateral *inguinal* herniae are uncommon in girls. This should be an alert to determine the peripheral karyotype. This had not been performed in the older sibling when she was first seen at age 18 months. Both sisters were 46 XY and androgen-receptor negative. This is the classical complete testicular feminization syndrome. Inheritance is X-linked. Presentation usually occurs in adult life because of primary amenorrhoea.

In this case, the herniae were troublesome. Bilateral repairs were performed with resiting of the gonads into the peritoneal cavity. Breast development will then occur spontaneously at the time of puberty; both affected siblings will require bilateral orchidectomy postpuberty, followed by oestrogen therapy.

7. DIAGNOSIS: PARTIAL ANDROGEN INSENSITIVITY SYNDROME ANDROGEN-RECEPTOR POSITIVE

CASE HISTORY

A mother was concerned that bilateral groin lumps had appeared in her 7-month-old daughter. The pregnancy had been normal and there was no relevant family history.

Examination showed mild cliteromegaly and a single orifice on the perineum. The labia majora were slightly rugose. Gonads measuring 3 ml in volume were palpable in both inguinal regions.

INVESTIGATIONS AND RESULTS

- Peripheral karyotype 46 XY
- Perineal sinogram: Contrast medium outlined a 'cavity' which was either a urogenital sinus or a blind-ending vagina

RESULTS

- Short HCG stimulation test
    2000 units i.m. daily for 3 days.

Steroid	Pre-HCG	Post-HCG	Units
17OH-Progesterone	8·0	9·2	nmol/l
Androstenedione	0·9	2·4	nmol/l
Testosterone	1·2	23·2	nmol/l
Dihydrotestosterone	0·41	0·76	nmol/l
T : DHT ratio	3·1	31·3	—
Oestradiol	41	172	pmol/l

● 24-h urinary steroids (measured by gas chromatography)
  normal for age
  No evidence of 5α-reductase enzyme deficiency

● Androgen receptors in genital skin fibroblasts
  Receptor concentration 727×10^{-18}mol/µg DNA   (*normal*)
  Binding affinity $0·63 \times 10^{-10}$M   (*normal*)
  Thermolabile at 40°C   (*abnormal*)
  Increased rate of dissociation   (*abnormal*)
  No augmentation with androgens   (*abnormal*)

COMMENT

This infant had male pseudohermaphroditism with severe incomplete masculinization. There was a marked testosterone response to HCG stimulation; this result and the karyotype indicated that the inguinal lumps were probably testes. Normal plasma levels of androstenedione excluded 17β-hydroxysteroid dehydrogenase deficiency. The ratio of testosterone (T) to dihydrotestosterone (DHT) following HCG stimulation was slightly elevated suggesting 5α-reductase deficiency. However, detailed profile of the urinary steroid metabolites excluded this diagnosis.

At operation, distinctly separate vaginal and urethral orifices were visualized on the perineum. Bilateral testes were found through inguinal incisions. The pelvis was explored through one of these incisions; no uterus, cervix, fallopian tubes or ovaries were found. Bilateral orchidectomy and a partial clitoral recession were performed. Histology of the gonads showed appearances of testes normal for an infant male. Genital skin fibroblasts were established in culture from clitoral skin. While there was a normal concentration of androgen receptors, detailed additional studies showed that androgen-receptor binding was qualitatively abnormal. Presumably this was due to a structural abnormality of the receptor protein causing a failure to respond to androgens. She will require oestrogen therapy later to induce puberty and also a vaginoplasty. This case is a variant of the testicular feminization syndrome.

8. DIAGNOSIS: AMBIGUOUS GENITALIA
MIXED GONADAL DYSGENESIS

CASE HISTORY

Full-term infant born following a normal pregnancy. Abnormal external genitalia noted. No relevant family history. There was a phallus 2 cm in length, rugose labioscrotal folds and a single urogenital opening on the perineum. A mass was palpable in the right groin.

INVESTIGATIONS AND RESULTS

- Plasma 17OH-progesterone 5 nmol/l
- Peripheral karyotype
     Mosaic 45 XO (28 per cent): 46 XY (72 per cent)
     No. of mitoses counted 76
- Intravenous pyelogram–*normal*
- Perineal sinogram—*uterus cavity demonstrated*
- Basal serum
     LH   11·2 U/l
     FSH   16·0 U/l
- Plasma
     Testosterone   8 nmol/l
- HCG stimulation (2000 units i.m. daily for 3 days)
     Plasma testosterone post-HCG 25·6 nmol/l.

COMMENT

Congenital adrenal hyperplasia due to 21-hydroxylase deficiency was excluded. The peripheral karyotype suggested mixed gonadal dysgenesis. At laparotomy there was a left streak ovary attached to a normal fallopian tube. On the right side there was an ovotestis. A normal uterus was present. Bilateral gonadectomy and clitoral recession was performed and the infant reared as a female. The karyotype was confirmed in cultures of clitoral skin and the right gonad.

9. DIAGNOSIS: DELAYED PUBERTY (FEMALE) RADIATION-INDUCED PRIMARY OVARIAN FAILURE

CASE HISTORY

An abdominal ganglion neuroblastoma was excised at age 12 months. Irradiation (3000 rad) was given to the abdomen because of residual islands of malignant tissue. At 15·2 years she was short and had delayed puberty. Her height was 138·8 cm ($-3·76$ s.d.). Breast development and pubic hair were Tanner stages 1 and 2, respectively. She was premenarchal. Bone age was 12·8 years.

INVESTIGATIONS AND RESULTS

● LHRH stimulation
    100 μg

Time min	LH U/l	FSH U/l	Oestradiol pmol/l
0	> 50	> 40	24
30	> 50	> 40	—
60	> 50	> 40	—
120	> 50	> 40	43

● Basal
    TSH 0·6 mU/l
    FT_4 14 pmol/l

COMMENT

This girl has primary ovarian failure based on low plasma oestradiol and elevated basal serum LH and FSH concentrations. The cause is radiation damage to the ovaries during infancy at a time when there is evidence of gonadotrophin-dependent growth and maturation of follicles. Pubic hair growth was stimulated by the production of adrenal androgens (adrenarche). Oestrogen replacement has been started to induce breast development; later a cyclical oestrogen : progestogen preparation will be required.

10. DIAGNOSIS: ACUTE MYELOID LEUKAEMIA
SECONDARY LYMPHOMA
RADIATION-INDUCED PRIMARY
OVARIAN FAILURE

CASE HISTORY

Presented at age 11 years with spontaneous bruising and purpura. Diagnosis of acute myeloid leukaemia established. After remission, she was treated with total body irradiation and an allogeneic bone marrow transplant. She subsequently developed a cerebral lymphoma which was totally excised. Cranial irradiation was given post-operatively. At age 14·0 years she was prepubertal. Her height was 151·5 cm (− 0·9 s.d.).

INVESTIGATIONS AND RESULTS

- Combined LHRH and TRH stimulation tests
  LHRH 100 μg i.v.
  TRH 200 μg i.v.

Time min	LH U/l	FSH U/l	TSH mU/l	Oestradiol pmol/l	T_4 nmol/l	T_3 nmol/l
0	> 50	> 40	2·0	< 20	101	2·4
30	> 50	> 40	12·3	—	—	—
60	> 50	> 40	8·1	—	—	—
120	> 50	> 40	4·5	< 20	110	3·0

- Short ACTH stimulation test
  Synacthen 250 μg i.m.

Time min	Plasma cortisol nmol/l	Plasma 17OHP nmol/l
0	147	0·9
60	900	6·5

COMMENT

As anticipated, whole body irradiation had caused complete ovarian failure. There was no evidence of thyroid dysfunction and the adrenal response to ACTH stimulation was entirely normal. Ethinyl oestradiol was given to induce breast development.

11. DIAGNOSIS: PREMATURE THELARCHE

CASE HISTORY

Female referred at 2 years because of breast development. Was a full-term, breast-fed infant. There was neonatal gynaecomastia which had persisted. Mother had been taking a progestogen-only oral contraceptive. There was bilateral true breast tissue, no pubic hair and a normal vaginal introitus. The cervix was palpable on rectal examination but there were no adnexal masses. Height, weight and head circumference were between 10th and 25th centiles.

INVESTIGATIONS AND RESULTS

- Bone age 1·6 years
- Pelvic ultrasound *normal*
- Plasma oestradiol 24 pmol/l
- Serum
LH	1·1 U/l
FSH	2·4 U/l
β-HCG	6·0 U/l

COMMENT

Breast development was isolated and unassociated with either rapid growth or advanced skeletal maturation. There was no known exposure to exogenous oestrogens. Rectal examination and pelvic ultrasound excluded an ovarian mass. Basal oestradiol and gonadotrophin levels were prepubertal. A normal HCG level ruled out the rare possibility of a primitive chorionic tumour. Premature thelarche is a benign condition; the exact cause is unknown.

12. DIAGNOSIS: PREMATURE THELARCHE

CASE HISTORY

Referred at age 4·5 years because of early breast development. This had been present since birth. She was receiving no medications. Her height was 111·2 cm (+ 1·6 s.d.). Breast development was Tanner stage 2; there was no pubic hair growth. The external genitalia were normal. No pelvic mass was palpable on rectal examination. Bone age was 7·1 years.

INVESTIGATIONS AND RESULTS
- Pelvic ultrasound *normal*
- LHRH stimulation test
  100 μg i.v.

Time min	LH U/l	FSH U/l	Oestradiol pmol/l
0	< 0·7	< 0·4	28
30	7·7	12·7	—
60	5·7	14·6	—
120	4·2	14·5	42

COMMENT

Signs of puberty were isolated to breast development only. However, bone age was significantly advanced and the gonadotrophin response (particularly FSH) to LHRH stimulation was exaggerated. These results suggested that breast development was the forerunner to true precocious puberty. During the next 6 months her growth velocity was 9·6 cm/year (> 97th centile). However, no other signs of puberty developed and by age 8·4 years there had been complete regression of breast development. It is possible that she developed a transient ovarian cyst, although this was never verified with ultrasound examinations.

13. DIAGNOSIS: IDIOPATHIC HIRSUTISM

CASE HISTORY

A girl aged 13·5 years was referred with a 10-month history of increased body hair. Menarche was at 11·5 years. Her menses were irregular. She was obese and had a normal blood pressure. She had hirsutism affecting the upper lip, chin, chest, thighs and legs. There was no acne. The external genitalia were normal.

INVESTIGATIONS

- Basal serum
    - LH
    - FSH
- Short ACTH stimulation
    - Synacthen 250 μg i.m.
- Overnight dexamethasone suppression
    - Dexamethasone 1 mg orally
- Pelvic ultrasound

RESULTS

- Basal serum
    - LH   11·1 U/l
    - FSH   4·9 U/l
- Plasma steroids

Time min	Cortisol nmol/l	17OH-Progesterone nmol/l	Androstenedione nmol/l	Testosterone nmol/l
Synacthen				
0	238	2·6	5·2	1·3
60	614	9·3	8·9	1·5
Clock time				
Dexamethasone				
24:00	50	2·5	—	—
08:00	< 28	1·1	< 3·6	1·1

- Pelvic ultrasound—*normal ovarian size*

COMMENT

In the absence of acne, hypertension and clitoromegaly, late-onset congenital adrenal hyperplasia or an adrenal tumour were unlikely causes for the hirsutism. Basal and ACTH-stimulated plasma concentrations of cortisol, and precursor steroids were normal. A defect in adrenal biosynthesis was excluded. Basal plasma testosterone concentration was normal for a postmenarchal female. Overnight dexamethasone caused complete suppression of adrenal biosynthesis. Normal ovaries demonstrated on ultrasound probably excluded polycystic ovarian disease (Stein–Leventhal syndrome). Treatment was started with a cyclical oestrogen : progesterone preparation and depilatory creams.

CHAPTER 7

The Endocrine Pancreas

In children, disorders of the endocrine pancreas produce either hyperglycaemia (i.e. diabetes mellitus) or hypoglycaemia. There has been an explosion in discovery and measurement recently of gut-related hormones. Conditions associated with increased production of these hormones, generally termed 'apudomas', are now being characterized. However, these are uncommon in children; since they usually present with symptoms and signs referable to the gastrointestinal tract, the appropriate investigations are not covered in this Handbook.

HYPERGLYCAEMIA

BASAL INVESTIGATIONS
- Fasting blood glucose
    - Venous whole blood
    - Capillary whole blood
    - Plasma
- 2-h postprandial blood glucose
- Serum ketones
- Glycosylated haemoglobin (HbA_1)
- Fructosamine
- Urine for glucose
    - 2-drop method (0–5 per cent glycosuria)
    - 5-drop method (0–2 per cent glycosuria)
  Tests available as Clinitest tablets or Clinistix and Diastix paper strips
- Urine for ketones
  Tests available as Acetest tablets, Ketostix and Ketodiastix
- Overnight urine for microalbuminuria
- Whole blood glucose on paper strips, e.g. Dextrostix, Visidex, B–M glycaemic strip.
    Interpretation: The fasting whole blood glucose or plasma glucose does not normally exceed 7–8 mmol/l. However, the

result *must* be interpreted relative to a venous or capillary blood sample, and to glucose determination in whole blood or plasma. Blood samples must be collected into tubes containing fluoride (unless paper strips are used). The method for determining glycosylated haemoglobin varies widely. The major component is termed HBA_1C, but many centres determine the total HbA_1. Normal range is approximately 5·0–8·5 per cent of total haemoglobin.

DYNAMIC INVESTIGATIONS

Oral Glucose Tolerance Test

● Ensure that the child has an adequate diet for at least 5 *days* before the test; in particular a *minimum* of 150 g/day of carbohydrate should be consumed
● Patient to be fasted
● Collect baseline blood sample for plasma glucose and serum insulin, and a urine sample for glucose and ketones ($t = 0$ min)
● Give a glucose solution orally; dose 1·75 g/kg up to a maximum of 75 g; the drink should be consumed in 5–10 min
● Collect blood samples for glucose and insulin at $t = 30, 60, 90$ and 120 min; occasionally further samples at 3, 4, 5 h are required
● Collect urine sample for glucose and ketones at 120 min.
    Interpretation: The entire profile of plasma glucose and insulin levels should be plotted graphically. However, an elevated fasting plasma glucose and a 2-h value exceeding 11 mmol/l is diagnostic of diabetes mellitus. Insulin values are quite variable in normals and may not provide any further diagnostic information. The results may indicate the degree of insulin reserve.

Intravenous Glucose Tolerance Test

● This test is rarely indicated in children
● 25 per cent glucose i.v. infusion over 5 min; dose 0·5 g/kg body weight
● Blood samples for glucose collected at 0, 10, 15, 20, 30 min.
    Interpretation: The disappearance rate of glucose is calculated by plotting plasma glucose values on a semilogarithmic scale against time. The disappearance rate is calculated ($t_{1/2}$) and used to calculate K, a rate constant, as follows:

$$K \text{ (rate constant for glucose)} = \frac{0 \cdot 693}{t_{1/2}} \times 100$$

The K value is usually less than 1 per cent in diabetic patients.

Note Most, if not all, children with diabetes do not require a glucose tolerance test to establish the diagnosis. A random plasma glucose is invariably > 11 mmol/l. Occasionally a child may develop transient hyperglycaemia and glycosuria during an intercurrent illness (usually an infection). In this instance, an OGTT is indicated to assess pancreatic β-cell reserve. But, the test must only be performed when the child has fully recovered and is eating an adequate diet.

HYPOGLYCAEMIA

In all age groups, apart from in the neonatal period, hypoglycaemia is defined as a blood glucose less than 2·2 mmol/l (40 mg/dl). Early neonatal hypoglycaemia which is transient usually occurs in low-birth-weight infants and will not be discussed further. Persistent symptomatic hypoglycaemia which is spontaneous requires urgent investigation and management. Appropriate investigation depends on the age group.

EARLY INFANCY

Basal investigations
- Blood glucose—performed on several occasions to confirm hypoglycaemia
- Plasma insulin—indicates if hyperinsulinism is the cause
- Serum ketones—distinguishes ketotic from non-ketotic hypoglycaemia
- Plasma pH, bicarbonate, lactate—possible inborn error of metabolism
- Serum GH   ⎫   possible deficiency of
  Plasma cortisol   ⎬ — counter-regulatory hormones
  Plasma catecholamines ⎭   as the cause.
- Urine ketones—as for serum ketones
- Urine-reducing substances, i.e. positive clinitest/negative clinistix—inborn error of carbohydrate metabolism, such as galactosaemia.

    Interpretation: Much information about the possible cause of hypoglycaemia can be obtained from a *single* blood sample collected at the time of hypoglycaemia with *carefully* selected investigations performed on the sample. Persistent neonatal hypoglycaemia is usually associated with hyperinsulinism due to pancreatic β-cell hyperplasia. The characteristic findings are:

- Persistently low blood glucose (< 2 mmol/l)
- Inappropriately elevated plasma insulin for low blood glucose level
- Increased insulin : glucose ratio
- Absent serum and urinary ketones
- Normal plasma pH, bicarbonate and lactate
- Appropriate elevation in serum GH, plasma cortisol and catecholamines in response to hypoglycaemic-induced stress.

An additional useful diagnostic pointer to hyperinsulinism is to calculate the amount of glucose required to maintain the blood glucose > 2 mmol/l. Glucose infusion rates 10–12 mg/kg per min are consistent with hyperinsulinism.

Occasionally a deficiency of a counter-regulatory hormone such as GH or cortisol can present as hypoglycaemia. The appropriate investigations to confirm pituitary and/or adrenal insufficiency are discussed in the relevant sections of the Handbook.

Dynamic Investigations

These are rarely required for the investigation of hypoglycaemia in early infancy. The glucagon stimulation test is useful for the diagnosis of some inborn errors of metabolism (*see below*).

OLDER INFANTS AND CHILDREN

In this age group it is usually necessary to provoke a stimulus for hypoglycaemia—a prolonged fast. The test is designed to answer two questions:

Dose the child become hypoglycaemic on fasting?
If so, what is the likeliest cause?

Prolonged Fasting

- Test *must* be performed as an in-patient under close supervision
- Time of starting and length of fast depends on age of child and clinical history.
  Infants 2 years—fast for 6–8 h
  Children 2–10 years—fast for 8–16 h
  Children > 10 years—fast for 16–20 h
  NB Can include overnight hours to start the fast in older children

- Weigh the child at start of fast
- Collect baseline blood and urine samples for glucose and ketones
- Monitor progress 2–4 hourly with capillary blood glucose (Dextrostix, B–M glycaemic etc.) and urine ketones
- Weigh the child after 6–12 h fasting
- If hypoglycaemia develops, collect blood samples immediately for glucose, ketones, *insulin,* lactate, GH and cortisol—then stop the test and give glucose
- If hypoglycaemia does not develop, stop fast at appropriate time for age (*see above*) and collect blood samples for above investigations before giving glucose
- Weigh the child at end of fast

    Interpretation: The prolonged fast is a useful screening procedure for suspected hypoglycaemic symptoms. Most children maintain normoglycaemia after an *appropriate* fast. If fasting is too prolonged, even normal children can become hypoglycaemic.

    As with the investigations described for newborn infants, an inappropriate increase in plasma insulin when the blood glucose is low indicates hyperinsulinism. In the older child, this is more likely to be caused by a pancreatic islet cell adenoma. Occasionally the diagnosis of primary adrenal insufficiency, GH or ACTH deficiency can be discovered during a prolonged fast.

Glucagon Stimulation Test

- Patient to be fasted; if there is spontaneous hypoglycaemia, the test can be performed to assess the response to glucagon during hypoglycaemia
- Collect baseline blood samples for glucose and insulin
- Give glucagon 0·1 mg/kg body weight i.m. (up to maximum 1 mg)
- Collect blood samples for glucose and insulin at 5, 10, 15, 20, 30, 60 min
- *Warning* There may be late, reactive hypoglycaemia if hyperinsulinism is present.

    Interpretation: An exaggerated insulin response (peak insulin level > 80 mU/l) suggests hyperinsulinism. In the older child and adult, this is likely to be due to an islet cell adenoma. There is also an increase in blood glucose levels, even in the presence of basal hypoglycaemia. An absent glycaemic response occurs with disorders of hepatic glycogen metabolism. The further investigations of inborn errors of carbohydrate metabolism are not discussed in this Handbook.

Leucine Tolerance Test

Patient to be fasted
Collect baseline blood samples for glucose and insulin
Give leucine 150 mg/kg body weight orally
Collect blood samples for glucose and insulin at 15, 30, 60, 90 min

Interpretation: Some children with hypoglycaemia are particularly sensitive to leucine, showing a marked fall in blood glucose and a rise in insulin levels. It is likely that this is just another index of hyperinsulinism rather than a specific entity associated with leucine sensitivity of the islet cell alone.

Tolbutamide Stimulation Test

Tolbutamide stimulates insulin release. The test is used occasionally in adults for the diagnosis of an islet cell adenoma. This investigation is potentially dangerous and is *not* recommended in children.

Other Investigations

Proinsulin—islet cell adenomas may secrete proinsulin predominantly.

C-peptide—is part of the connecting chain which remains intact during the conversion of proinsulin to insulin. Since it is secreted in equimolar amounts with insulin, it is a useful marker of β-cell function. Insulin and C-peptide measurements are independent of each other when determined by radioimmunoassay. For example, it is possible to assess β-cell response to glucose in a diabetic patient receiving exogenous insulin. In the context of suspected hypoglycaemia, C-peptide measurements can be valuable to document surreptitious exogenous insulin administration. Typically, the following are observed:

Low blood glucose levels
Elevated insulin levels
● Lack of temporal relation to fasting
Absent ketones in serum and urine
Suppressed C-peptide levels.

CASE ILLUSTRATIONS

1. Persistent neonatal hypoglycaemia
   Nesidioblastosis
2. Insulin-dependent diabetes mellitus
3. Severe diabetic ketoacidosis
   Hyperlipaemia

1. DIAGNOSIS: PERSISTENT NEONATAL HYPOGLYCAEMIA NESIDIOBLASTOSIS

CASE HISTORY

A female infant, birth weight 3990 g, was born at 40 weeks gestation to a primigravida mother. Pregnancy was normal. The immediate neonatal period was uneventful. On day 4, she had a severe apnoeic episode. Her blood sugar was 0·6 mmol/l; there was a dramatic response to intravenous glucose. She later had a major fit which required intravenous phenobarbitone. Lumbar puncture was normal.

INVESTIGATIONS AND RESULTS
- Serum calcium 2·44 mmol/l (N 2·25–2·60)
- Plasma
  Lactate 1·00 mmol/l (N 0·63–2·44)
  Pyruvate 25 μmol/l (*normal*)
- RBC galactose-1-phosphate uridyl transferase *normal*
- Plasma and urinary amino acids *normal*
- Urine ketones *negative*
- Plasma hormone profiles during hypoglycaemia:

Glucose mmol/l	Insulin mU/l	C-peptide pmol/ml	GH mU/l	Cortisol nmol/l
1·8	22·5	1·4	19·4	580
0·7	38·4	1·5	—	—
1·2	19·0	0·88	—	—

Glucose infusion rate to maintain euglycaemia: 14 mg/kg per min (normal 6–8).

COMMENT

The apnoeic episode was due to hypoglycaemia. There were no predisposing factors during pregnancy. The hypoglycaemia was severe, persistent and non-ketotic. The cause of the hypoglycaemia was established on the basis of inappropriately elevated concentrations of insulin and C-peptide at the time of hypoglycaemia. There was no deficiency of counter-regulatory hormones such as GH and cortisol. Prior to surgery, a large glucose infusion rate was required to offset the effect of hyperinsulinism. This in itself is a useful diagnostic test.

A 95 per cent subtotal pancreatectomy was performed. Histology showed diffuse islet cell hyperplasia consistent with nesidioblastosis. Exogenous insulin replacement was required for 2 weeks postoperatively. Random capillary blood glucose measurements were satisfactory while she was fed 4-hourly. Four weeks following surgery, the pancreatic β-cell response to an oral glucose load (1·75 g/kg) was measured:

Time min	Plasma glucose mmol/l	Insulin mU/l	C-peptide pmol/ml
0	4·3	10	0·21
30	4·9	18	0·84
60	6·2	26	0·72
90	6·2	15	0·55
120	7·2	20	0·69

Fasting plasma glucose was normal. There is some residual islet cell function and no evidence for recurrence of hyperinsulinism. Continued profiles of capillary blood glucose levels are required. Her development is satisfactory, although there is some hypotonia.

2. DIAGNOSIS: INSULIN-DEPENDENT DIABETES MELLITUS

CASE HISTORY

A boy aged 12 years presented with a 4-week history of polydipsia and polyuria. He was always hungry and lost weight. He had frequent episodes of tonsillitis. There was no relevant family history. He looked thin, but was not dehydrated or acidotic.

INVESTIGATIONS AND RESULTS

- Plasma

Glucose	33·6 mmol/l
Urea	5·9 mmol/l
Na	130 mmol/l
K	4·2 mmol/l

- pH   7·34

Bicarbonate	21·4 mmol/l
Base deficit	− 4·1 mmol/l

- Urinalysis

  Glucose 4+
  Ketones large

COMMENT

The history was typical for diabetes mellitus. Symptoms are present for a short duration in children. He was not dehydrated or ketoacidotic. However he had hyponatraemia; this did not require intravenous saline for correction. When the plasma glucose concentration was reduced with insulin therapy, a repeat plasma sodium 12 h later was normal (138 mmol/l). There was no evidence of hyperlipidaemia which could cause a spurious decrease in sodium concentration. In this case, the mechanism is probably due to hyperglycaemia promoting both an osmotic diuresis and an osmotic shift of water from within the cells to the extracellular fluid. This decreases the plasma sodium concentration by dilution. Thus if there is no dehydration or ketoacidosis, intravenous saline is not required to correct hyponatraemia.

3. DIAGNOSIS: **SEVERE DIABETIC**
                          KETOACIDOSIS HYPERLIPAEMIA

CASE HISTORY

A girl aged 7 years was admitted to hospital as an emergency. She had been acutely ill for 24 hours with rapid breathing, vomiting and feeling cold. There was a 3–4 week history of polydipsia, polyuria, voracious appetite and recent weight loss. She was severely dehydrated, hypothermic and was hyperventilating. The peripheral circulation was poor.

INVESTIGATIONS AND RESULTS

- Plasma

Glucose	18·1 mmol/l	
Urea	2·8 mmol/l	
Na	81 mmol/l	
K	2·1 mmol/l	
pH	6·94	(N 7·36–7·44)
PO_2	51 mmHg	(N 90–110)
PCO_2	23 mmHg	(N 22–27)
Bicarbonate	7·7 mmol/l	(N 22–27)
Base deficit	31·9	(N −3 to +3)

- Hyperlipaemic serum
- Salicylate screen *negative.*

COMMENT

This girl had acute onset insulin-dependent diabetes mellitus and severe ketoacidosis. The degree of hyponatraemia was spuriously altered by the effect of lipaemic serum on electrolyte determinations. She was resuscitated with plasma expanders, normal saline, intravenous bicarbonate and a continuous low-dose infusion of insulin. She made an uneventful recovery and is currently controlled on a twice daily insulin regimen. In a subsequent fasting blood sample collected when she was well, plasma triglyceride and cholesterol concentrations were normal.

CHAPTER 8

The Molecular Biology of Endocrine Disease

It is appropriate to include a brief chapter in the Handbook on the potential application of the techniques of molecular biology to the investigation of endocrine diseases in children. Several inherited endocrine disorders are recognised in childhood, particularly involving adrenal, thyroid and gonadal function. A vast array of cDNA probes are now available to study the human genome and several endocrine disorders can be investigated by nucleic acid hybridization analysis. The clinical investigator is the most important initial cog in the long chain of events that starts with DNA extraction and finishes typically with the procedure of Southern blotting and autoradiography. The details of the techniques are beyond the scope of this Handbook but it is important that the clinician is competent to know (a) which samples to collect for DNA analysis and (b) which endocrine disorders can be investigated by recombinant DNA technology.

SAMPLES

- *Blood* Collect sample into EDTA tubes and transfer immediately to laboratory for best results. Whole blood samples can be stored frozen until transferred to the laboratory but must be transported on dry ice to avoid thawing. Sample volume ideally 20 ml blood, but 2–3 ml from infants is acceptable. Yield of DNA is dependent on sample volume and white cell count. Newer techniques now allow enough DNA to be extracted from blood spots. Ensure blood samples are obtained from all appropriate family members.

● *Fibroblasts* This is another useful source of DNA. Do *not* freeze cells until cultures are harvested.

  Organ-specific tissues —Liver
                                   —brain
                                   —spleen
                                   —adrenals
                                   —chorionic villi

Tissues can be stored frozen until DNA extracted.

ENDOCRINE DISORDERS

The following is a list of some endocrine disorders of childhood which are amenable to investigation using appropriate cDNA probes:

Isolated GH deficiency (familial type IA).

Laron dwarfism (IGF-I deficiency).

Congenital adrenal hyperplasia (particularly 21-hydroxylase deficiency).

Testicular feminisation syndrome.

Placental sulphatase deficiency.

Vitamin D resistant rickets.

● Familial ADH deficiency.

Multiple endocrine neoplasia syndrome.

● Prader-Willi Syndrome.

APPENDIX

NORMAL VALUES

The following serves only as a guide to normal ranges for some hormone concentrations. Results differ according to assay methods and between laboratories. For some hormones, no normal range has yet been established for children, particularly in young infants. The clinician should discuss the interpretation of the results of endocrine tests with laboratory staff if necessary.

When appropriate, the Appendix contains normal ranges expressed also in Traditional Units as shown in parentheses. Conversion factors have not been applied to polypeptide hormone values as their measurement is entirely dependent on the standards used in the assay. For example, LH and FSH are either measured using NIBSC material (National Institute of Biological Standards and Controls) which are International Reference Preparations (IRP) or by standards provided by the National Institutes of Health (NIH, Bethesda). The latter measured in Traditional Units (e.g. ng/ml) can be expressed as equivalent to units of the IRP.

PITUITARY

GH	—Basal value low, often undetectable —Peak value > 15 mU/l after appropriate stimulation	
ACTH	—Basal value 10–80 ng/l at 09:00 h	

TSH	—Basal < 5 mU/l
	—Peak value following TRH stimulation:
	     Mean ± s.d. 12·3± 3·2 mU/l
	     Range 5·4 – 25·0 mU/l	

PRL	—Basal < 420 mU/l	
LH	—Basal	
	Prepubertal	0·6 – 1·7 U/l
	Pubertal	0·8 – 8·7 U/l
	Follicular	3·0 – 12·0 U/l
	Mid-cycle	25 – 64 U/l
	Luteal	2·4 – 13·0 U/l
	Postmenopausal	29 – 120 U/l
	—Peak value following LHRH stimulation	
	Prepubertal: Mean ± s.d.	3·9±1·9 U/l
	Range	1·5 – 11·9 U/l
	Pubertal*: Mean ± s.d.	21·7±2·9 U/l
	Range	5·9 – 48·8 U/l
FSH	—Basal	
	Prepubertal	0·6 – 3·4 U/l
	Pubertal*	0·6 – 4·9 U/l
	Follicular	2·0 – 6·6 U/l
	Mid-cycle	—
	Luteal	1·6 – 5·7 U/l
	Postmenopausal	28 – 130 U/l
	—Peak value following LHRH stimulation	
	Prepubertal: Mean ± s.d.	3·9±5·6 U/l
	Range	1·5 – 10·8 U/l
	Pubertal*: Mean ± s.d.	4·1±1·4 U/l
	Range	2·2 – 8·0 U/l
ADH	—Basal 1 – 5 pmol/l; not routinely available	
Plasma osmolality	—275 – 295 mOsm/kg H_2O (*see* p. 18)	

*These data were derived from a group of boys and girls who were in puberty (stages 2–5) and had a bone age > 12·5 years. More detailed data are reported in the literature for males and females separately and for different stages of puberty.[1, 2].

THYROID

Total T_4	55–150 nmol/l	(4–12 μg/dl)
Total T_3	1·2–3·1 nmol/l	(78–200 ng/dl)
FT_4	8–26 pmol/l	(0·6–2·0 ng/dl)
FT_3	3–9 pmol/l	(0·19–0·59 ng/dl)
TSH	< 5 mU/l	
TBG	12–31 ng/l	
Tg	< 60 ng/ml	
Serum carotene	0·6–2·1 μmol/l	(32–113 μg/dl)
TSH receptor antibodies	−10 to +10 per cent inhibition of binding	
^{123}I uptake	10–40 per cent uptake at 4 h	
ETR	0·86–1·13	
Perchlorate discharge	< 10 per cent at 1 h	

CALCIUM, PARATHYROID, VITAMIN D

Calcium	2·26–2·80 mmol/l	(9–11 mg/dl)
Phosphate	0·80–1·45 mmol/l	(2·5–4·5 mg/dl)
Magnesium	0·7–1·2 mmol/l	(1·7–2·9 mg/dl)
Sodium	133–144 mmol/l	(133–144 mEq/l)
Potassium	3·4–5·2 mmol/l	(3·4–5·2 mEq/l)
Chloride	95–105 mmol/l	(95–105 mEq/l)
Bicarbonate	22–30 mmol/l	(22–30 mEq/l)
Urea	2·5–7·5 mmol/l	(7–21 mg/dl)
Creatinine	60–120 μmol/l	(0·7–1·4 mg/dl)
Total protein	60–80 g/l	(6·0–8·0 g/dl)
Albumin	35–45 g/l	(3·5–4·5 g/dl)
Alkaline phosphatase	30–95 IU/l	
PTH	< 1·0 ng/ml	
25-HCC	8–50 ng/ml	
Calcitonin	< 0·08 ng/l	
Urine TMP/GFR	0·7–1·4 mmol/l	
TMCa/GFR	1·6–2·1 mmol/l	

ADRENAL CORTEX

Plasma	ACTH	10–80 ng/l	
	Cortisol	140–800 nmol/l	(5–29 µg/dl)
	17-OHP	< 15 nmol/l	(< 45 ng/dl)
	11-Deoxycortisol	< 60 nmol/l	
	Androstenedione		
	Children	< 3·6 nmol/l	
	Male	4·4–10·6 nmol/l	
	Female	4·0–10·2 nmol/l	
Urine:	Urinary free cortisol	< 350 nmol/day	(13 µg/day)
	17-Oxosteroids		
	Infants	< 3 µmol/day	(0·9 mg/day)
	Children	< 12 µmol/day	(3·5 mg/day)
	Pregnanetriol		
	Infants	< 0·3 µmol/day	(< 0·1 mg/day)
	Children	< 3 µmol/day	(< 1 mg/day)
	11-Oxygenation index	< 0·7	

Note: Many of these urinary steroid measurements have been superseded by more detailed analysis of urinary adrenocortical metabolites as measured by high-pressure liquid chromatographic (HPLC) and mass spectrometry–gas chromatographic (GC–MS) techniques. These are only available in specialized laboratories.

ADRENAL MEDULLA

24-h urinary VMA	< 35 µmol/day	(< 7 mg/day)
24-h urinary metadrenaline	< 6·5 µmol/day	

Note: These values should also be expressed in relation to urinary creatinine excretion.

GONADS

LH/FSH		
—*see under* pituitary		
Plasma testosterone		
Prepubertal	< 0·5 nmol/l	(< 15 ng/dl)
Adult female	·3–2·5 nmol/l	(9–70 ng/dl)
Adult male	10–30 nmol/l	(300–900 ng/dl)
Plasma oestradiol		
Prepubertal	< 60 pmol/l	(< 16 pg/ml)
Adult male	< 250 pmol/l	(< 68 pg/ml)
Follicular	70–260 pmol/l	(19–70 pg/ml)
Mid-cycle	350–1500 pmol/l	(95–405 pg/ml)
Luteal	180–1100 pmol/l	(49–297 pg/ml)
Postmenopausal	< 250 pmol/l	(< 68 pg/ml)
Plasma progesterone		
Prepubertal	< 1·3 nmol/l	(< 40 ng/dl)
Adult male	< 1·3 nmol/l	(< 40 ng/dl)
Follicular	0·3–4·8 nmol/l	(9–149 ng/dl)
Luteal	8·0–90 nmol/l	(248–2790 ng/dl)
Mid-luteal	18·3–90 nmol/l	(567–2790 ng/dl)
Postmenopausal	< 0·6 nmol/l	(< 19 ng/dl)

Note: Plasma sex steroid concentrations are different during early infancy as well as at each stage of puberty.[3]

ENDOCRINE PANCREAS

Plasma glucose (fasting)	2·8–6·5 mmol/l	(50–117 mg/dl)
Total HbA₁	5·7–8·0 per cent	
Plasma insulin*	< 10 mU/l	
Plasma C-peptide	0·2–0·6 pmol/l	

*Plasma insulin measurements must be interpreted in relation to concomitant plasma glucose values. Normally plasma insulin should not exceed 10 mU/l when the fasting plasma glucose concentration is normal or low.

References

1. Job J. C., Chaussain J. L. and Garnier P. E. (1977) The use of LHRH in paediatric patients. *Hormone Research,* **8,** 171–187.
2. Dickerman Z., Prager-Lewin R., and Laron Z. (1976) Response of plasma LH and FSH to synthetic LH-RH in children at various pubertal stages. *Am. J. Dis. Child.* **120,** 634–638.
3. Winter J. S. D. (1978) Prepubertal and pubertal endocrinology. In: *Human Growth, Vol. 2: Postnatal Growth.* Eds F. Falkner and J. M. Tanner. pp. 183–213. New York: Plenum Press.

INDEX

acromegaly 13
Addison's disease 76
  investigations 100, 101
  pigmentation 101
  thyroid autoantibodies 62
  treatment 102
adrenal cortex, hormone classes 83–94
  see also individual hormones, hormone
    classes
adrenalectomy 99
adrenal gland 83–109
  failure 101 see also Addison's disease
  insufficiency 87
    secondary 90
    Synacthen test 89, 90
  steroid biosynthesis scheme 86, 87
  steroid in plasma 87
adrenal medulla
  cathecholamines 94, 95
  enzymes 96
  investigations 96
  function tests 96
adrenal venogram 99
adrenocortical function tests
  glucocorticoids 85–94
  mineralocorticoids 92–96
adrenocorticotrophin (ACTH)
  dexamethasone suppression 16, 17
  diurnal rhythm 87
  ectopic syndrome 87
  insulin tolerance test 15
  metyrapone test 15, 16
  normal values 141, 143
  sampling 87, 89
  secretion control 15
  suppression tests, 16, 17, 90
  Synacthen stimulation 89, 90
  urinary metabolites 88, 89
    oxogenic or ketogenic steroids
      89
adverse reactions
  arginine 11
  clonidine 12
  L-Dopa 11
  metyrapone 16
  metoclopramide 12

adverse reactions (cont.)
  TSH stimulation 14
air encephalography 44
aldosterone
  secretion control 93
  structure 84
alopecia areata 69
ambiguous genitalia
  congenital adrenal hyperplasia 103,
    104, 114
  investigations, flow diagram 115, 124
    and management 124
amenorrhoea and hyperprolactinaemia
  114
cAMP, urinary 74, 82
androgen insensitivity syndrome 121,
  122
  gonad features 122, 123
  human chorionic gonadotrophin
    stimulation test 113
  partial 122, 123
  treatment 122, 123
androgen receptor binding 118, 119
  negative 121, 122
  positive 122, 123
androstenedione 110
  normal values 143
angiotensin 93
anosmia 52 see also Kallmann's
  syndrome
anovulation, conditions 114
antidiuretic hormone
  normal values 142
  water deprivation test 18
apnoea 137
apudomas 130
arginine stimulation test 11, 19, 20
  delayed puberty 22–23
    growth hormone deficiency 28, 30
  growth hormone deficiency 34–35
    and hydrocephalus 42, 43
  medulloblastoma radiotherapy 50,
    51
  pineal germinoma 48, 49
  septo-optic dysplasia 40
  short stature 58

147

auto-antibodies *see also* long-acting
thyroid stimulator
Addison's disease 101
Graves' disease 70, 71
Hashimoto's thyroiditis 68, 69
thyroid 62, 63, 102

blood
glucose tests 130, 131
monitoring 3
sample collection 3, 6
blood spots 3

calcitonin
auto-immune thyroiditis 69
in malignancy 77
normal values 142
pentagastrin stimulation test 77, 79
properties 76
provocative test 77
calcium metabolism 72–82
hypocalcaemia 72, 73
and protein concentration 73
calcium, normal values 142
carbimazole in Graves' disease 71
catecholamine synthesis and metabolism
scheme 94, 95
chorionic villus biopsy 107
cleft palate 32
congenital adrenal hyperplasia *see also*
11β-hydroxylase, 21-hydroxylase
ambiguous genitalia 103, 114, 115
treatment 104
case histories 102–107
causes and enzymes 87
investigations 102–107
late-onset, features 104–107
family screening 105–107
investigations 104, 105
treatment 108
male 102, 103
11-oxygenation index 89
salt-losing 102, 103
treatment 103
Conn's syndrome, investigations 94
corticotrophin-releasing factor 15
cotisol 10
diurnal secretion pattern 85
normal values 143
structure 84
urinary free 88

computerized tomography (CT) scan 42
panhypopituitarism 40, 41
C-peptide
and β-cell function 135
normal values 144
craniopharyngioma
necrotic 44
thyroid function 44
triple stimulation test 44, 45
creatine kinase test
false positive 66
in hypothyroidism 66
creatinine excretion 88
cryptorchidism 112
bilateral, investigation and treatment
117
Cushing's disease 87
dexamethasone suppression 98, 99
pituitary-dependent 98
investigations 98, 99
treatment 99
Cushing's syndrome 16, 17
adrenal tumour 87
investigation scheme 90, 92
urinary glucocorticoids 88
cyproterone acetate 55
cytochrome P450 107

DDAVP (1-desamino-8-D-arginine-
vasopressin)
and antidiuretic hormone test 18
diabetes insipidus test and control 56,
57
delayed puberty
female
hormone profiles 32, 33
investigations 125
radiation effects 125
treatment 125
male, case illustrations 22–31, 36, 37
growth hormone deficiency 36, 37
head injury 28–31
hormone profiles 23, 25
pubic hair 24
dexamethasone structure 85
dexamethasone suppression test
adrenocorticotrophin 16, 17, 90
Cushing's disease 98, 99
high-dose 17, 90
hirsutism 129
low-dose 17, 90
overnight 16, 90

diabetes insipidus 45
  central and head injury 56, 57
  control 57
  nephrogenic 18
  water deprivation test 56, 57
diabetes mellitus 16
  diagnosis in children 132
  insulin-dependent 64, 137, 138
    investigations 138
  osmotic diuresis 138
diabetic ketoacidosis
  investigations 138, 139
  treatment 139
dihydrotestosterone 110
DNA 107, 112, 140
  probes 107, 113, 140–141
Duchenne muscular dystrophy 66

electroencephalogram, sleep monitoring
  of growth hormone 9
Ellsworth-Howard test 74
endocrine tests, principles 1–7
  dynamic 1
  scheme 1, 2
  side effects 1 *see also* adverse reactions
exercise testing
  bicycle 9
  growth hormone 9

fasting
  duration 3
  and endocrine tests 1, 3
  and hypoglycaemia 133, 134
fludrocortisone structure 85
follicle stimulating hormone, normal
  values 141
food interfering with tests 3

galactosaemia 132
gas chromatography–mass spectrometry
  89
genitalia *see* ambiguous, micropenis
glucagon test
  congenital hypopituitarism, 38, 39
  growth hormone deficiency 40, 41
  hypoglycaemia 134, 135
  physiological effects 11
  septo-optic dysplasia 40, 41

glucocorticoids
  function tests 85–90
  normal values 143
glucose, normal plasma values 144
glucose tolerance test
  β-cell reserve 132
  disappearance rate 131
  intravenous 131, 132
  oral, procedure 131
glycosylated haemoglobin 131
goitre 67
gonadal dysgenesis, investigation and
  management 124
gonadotrophin deficiency 18
  pineal germinoma 48, 49
gonadotrophin-releasing hormone
  and gonadal function 18, 110
  test 18
gonads 110–129
  normal steroid hormone values 144
Graves' disease 62, 63
  auto-antibodies 70, 71
  clinical features 70
  family and case history 70
  thyroid scintigraphy 63
  T_3 suppression test 64
  treatment 71
growth hormone
  indications for testing 1
  normal values 141
  profile 9
  pulsatile secretion 9
  result spectrum 29
  secretion tests
    exercise 9, 58
    pharmacological 10–13
    physiological 8–10
    random 8
    sleep 9, 28, 58
  sleep and awake 9
  stimulation 8–13
    arginine 11, 19, 20
    clonidine 12
    L-Dopa 11, 12
    glucagon 11
    growth hormone-releasing hormone
      13
    insulin-induced 10, 11
    metoclopramide 12
  suppression 13
  synthetic 59
  treatment hazard 59
growth hormone deficiency
  definition 5, 6
  hormone profiles of isolated 34–35

growth hormone deficiency (*cont.*)
  hydrocephalus 42, 43
  partial and delayed puberty 36, 37
  pineal germinoma 48, 49
  radiation-induced 46, 47
  replacement 38, 40
  septo-optic dysplasia 40
growth hormone-releasing hormone
  congenital hypopituitarism 38, 39
  delayed puberty 28
    growth hormone deficiency 36, 37
  growth hormone testing 13
gut-related hormones 130
gynaecomastia
  investigations 120
  premature thelarche 127
  transient 121

Hashimoto's thyroiditis *see* thyroiditis,
    auto-immune
head injury
  and delayed puberty, male 28–31
  diabetes insipidus 56, 57
hernia, inguinal in girls 122
hirsutism, idiopathic 129
  features 128
  investigations 129
  treatment 129
HLA typing, congenital adrenal
    hyperplasia 104, 106, 107
homovanillic acid 95
hormone action scheme 1, 2
hormone measurements
  normal ranges 6, 141–144
  profile 5, 6
  techniques 5, 6
human chorionic gonadotrophin (HCG)
  ambiguous genitalia 115
  Leydig cell responses 119, 120
  micropenis 118, 119
  partial androgen insensitivity syndrome
    122, 123
  short-term, long-term tests in
    Kallmann's syndrome 52, 53
  stimulation in delayed puberty 26, 27
  testicular function 111, 112
    prolonged 112
hydrocephalus 41
  growth hormone deficiency 42, 43
  relief 43
hydrocortisone suppression test,
    hypercalcaemia 76

11β-hydroxylase deficiency 87, 115
  and action 86
  autosomal recessive 108
  congenital adrenal hyperplasia 107–109
    genitalia 107
    investigations 108
    treatment 108
    virilization 108
21-hydroxylase deficiency 87, 115
  action 86
  and congenital adrenal hyperplasia
    102–104
  diagnosis 89
  family screening 105, 107
  HLA linkage 106, 107
3 β-hydroxysteroid dehydrogenase
    deficiency 87, 104
  action 86
hyperaldosteronism *see* Conn's syndrome
hypercalcaemia *see also*
    hyperparathyroidism
  familial hypercalciuric 76
  investigations 75, 76
    dynamic 76
  phosphate clearance 75
hypercortisolism 90
hyperglycaemia
  investigations 130–132
  transient 132
hyperinsulinism 137
  diagnosis 133
hyperlipaemia 139
hyperparathyroidism
  and parathyroid adenoma tests 79
  thallium scan 79
hypertension, childhood 109
hyperthyroidism *see* Graves' disease
hypocalcaemia *see also* rickets
  investigations 72–75
    dynamic 74, 75
  renal function 73
hypoglycaemia
  blood sample use 132
  fasting in children 133
    prolonged 133, 134
    screening 134
    weight 134
  full-term infant 38
  glucagon stimulation test 134,
    135
  growth hormone measurement 10, 11
  intravenous glucose 36
  investigation 132–136
  leucine tolerance test 135
  persistent neonatal 136, 137

hypogonadism
  androgen replacement 116
  primary 112
  and testicular torsion 116
hypogonadotrophic hypogonadism *see*
    also Kallmann's syndrome
  luteinizing hormone releasing hormone
    stimulation 111
hypoparathyroidism *see also*
    hypocalcaemia
  investigations 74, 75
  phosphate and creatinine clearance
    74, 75
hypopituitarism, congenital
  case history 38
  investigations and hormonal response
    38, 39
hypothalamus 8, 17
  defect 38
  radiation damage 50
hypothyroidism 16
  congenital, thyroid tests 65, 66
  primary, thyroid tests 67, 68

immunoassays 5
insulin
  normal values 144
  variability 131
insulin-like growth factor I 9
insulin tolerance test
  adrenocorticotrophin test 15
  contraindications 10
  growth hormone deficiency 34–35
  growth hormone measurement 10, 11
iodine [^{123}I], uptake in autoimmune
    thyroiditis 68, 69 *see also* sodium
    iodide

Kallmann's syndrome
  definition 53
  family 53
  karyotype 52
  treatment 53
karyotype
  ambiguous genitalia 115, 124
  and testicular function 112
Klinefelter's syndrome 121

Laron dwarfism 142
LATS 63

leucine tolerance test, procedure 135
leukaemia, irradiation effects 126
Leydig cell function 26
long-acting thyroid stimulator (LATS) 63
luteinizing hormone, normal values 141
luteinizing hormone releasing hormone
    (LH–RH) *see also* triple
    stimulation test
  analogue, long-acting 55
  congenital hypopituitarism 38, 39
  delayed puberty 125
  gonadotrophin response 30
  Kallmann's syndrome 52
  precocious puberty response 54, 55
  testicular function test 111
lymphoma, cerebral 126

medulloblastoma, radiation damage 50,
    51
menstrual cycle, hormone profiles 113,
    114
metoclopramide stimulation 12
  delayed puberty 28
  radiation-induced growth hormone
    deficiency 46, 47
  in tests 12, 14
metyrapone test
  adrenocorticotrophin 15, 16
  exaggerated response 16
  mode of action 15
  short 16
micropenis 38, 52
  androgen receptors 118–120
  investigations 118, 119
  treatment 119, 120
mineralocorticoids
  and adrenal function tests 92–94
  biosynthesis 86, 92
multiple endocrine neoplasia syndrome,
  components 78

Nelson's syndrome 99
nesidioblastosis 136, 137
neuroblastoma 96
  radiation effects 125
nucleic acid hybridization analysis 140

obesity
  endocrine related 100
  plasma cortisol 100

oestradiol 110
  hypothalamus damage 50, 51
  menstrual cycle 113
  normal values 144
  structure 84
osmolality 31, 56
osteoporosis 77
ovarian failure 50
  investigations 126
  radiation-induced 125, 126
ovary
  function investigations 114
  steroids secreted 113
ovulation assessment 114

pancreas 130–139
pancreatectomy 137
pancreatic β-cell
  function after pancreatectomy 137
  hyperplasia 132
panhypopituitarism
  and septo-optic dysplasia 40, 41
  triple stimulation test 44, 45
parathyroid gland adenoma 79
parathyroid hormone
  hypercalcaemia 75
  normal values 142
  renal response test 74, 75
parathyroid function 72–82
Pendred's syndrome 67
pentagastrin stimulation test, calcitonin 77
pertechnetate ($^{99}Tc^{m}$) 63
phaeochromocytoma 96
  excision 109
  hypertension treatment 109
  investigations 96, 109
  noradrenaline 96
  size 96
phosphate
  clearance and reabsorption 74, 75
  excretion index 75
  normal values 142
  tubular maximum reabsorption 75
pineal germinoma, radiotherapy effects
  48, 49
pituitary gland *see also* hypothalamus
  anterior, hormones produced 8
  case illustrations 21–59
  endocrine testing 8–59
  gigantism 13
  normal hormone values 141
  posterior, hormones 8
  radiation damage 46
  triple stimulation test 19

placental sulphatase deficiency 141
Prader-Willi syndrome 141
precocious puberty 18
  idiopathic, female 54, 55
  treatment 55
prednisolone structure 84
pregnancy 114
pregnanetriol, normal values 143
premature thelarche
  benign, investigations 127, 128
  and bone age 128
preparation for tests 1, 6
  fasting 1, 3
primary gonadal failure 18
progesterone
  menstrual cycle 113
  normal values 142
  structure 84
17OH progesterone
  congenital adrenal hyperplasia
    102–104
  urinary metabolites 88, 89
proinsulin secretion 135
prolactin
  insulin tolerance test 10, 14
  normal values 141
  release stimulation 14
  secretion control 14
pseudohermaphroditism 123
  human chorionic gonadotrophin
    response 123
pseudohypoparathyroidism 75
  cAMP/creatinine ratio 82
  investigations 81
  parathyroid hormone 82
  treatment 81, 82

radiotherapy 46
  gonadotrophin deficiency 48, 49
  medulloblastoma 50, 51
  ovarian failure 125, 126
renal function tests 18, 74
renal tubule defects 80
renin-angiotensin system 92, 93
renin in congenital adrenal hyperplasia
  102, 103
restriction enzymes 107
rhabdomyosarcoma, pituitary effects of
  treatment 46
rickets
  classification and aetiology 73
  investigation 80
  vitamin D-dependent 73

rickets (*cont.*)
  vitamin D-resistant 73
    treatment 80
ring Y-chromosome anomaly 58, 59

saliva, sample collection 4
salt-losing states 92
samples *see also* individual fluids
  adrenocorticotrophin 87
  labelling 4, 7
  processing 4, 5, 7
sarcoidosis 76
Schmidt's syndrome 102
septo-optic dysplasia
  and growth hormone deficiency 40
  pituitary deficiencies 40
short stature 32
  extreme, investigations 58, 59
  karyotype 59
sodium balance studies 92, 94
  acute depletion 94
  and diet 94
sodium iodide [^{123}I] 63
  uptake and thyroid gland 63, 64
steroid nucleus structure 83
steroid synthesis
  inherited disorders 87
  scheme of adrenal 86
stress and prolactin release 10, 14
Sustanon components 10
Synacthen stimulation
  congenital adrenal hyperplasia 104,
    105
  congenital hypopituitarism, 38, 39
  hirsutism 129
  prolonged 90
  short, procedure 89

T$_3$ *see* trio-iodothyronine
T$_4$ *see* thyroxine
Tanner stages 110
testicular feminization syndrome 122
  partial androgen insensitivity 122, 123
testicular function 110–112
  failure 110
  intra-abdominal tissue 117
  karyotype 112
  tests 111–112
testicular prostheses 117
testicular torsion and atrophy 116
testis determining factor 112

testosterone
  biosynthesis pathway 110, 111
  human chorionic gonadotrophin test
    112
  levels and puberty 110
  normal values 144
  structure 84
thyroglobulin measurement 61–62
thyroid auto-antibodies 62, 71
thyroid carcinoma, medullary and
    calcitonin 77
  syndrome 78
thyroid function tests 44
thyroid gland 60–71
  biopsy 67
  definitive tests 62–64
  ectopic sublingual 66
  normal hormonal values 142
  organification defect 64
  replacement therapy 65
thyroiditis, auto-immune 67
  and alopecia 69
  antibodies and tests 68
  Hashimoto's 62, 68, 69
  iodine uptake 68, 69
thyroid profile components 60–62
  congenital hypothyroidism 65, 66
  primary hypothyroidism 67, 68
thyroid scintigraphy, isotopes used 63,
    64
thyroid-stimulating hormone (TSH)
  basal levels 14
  normal values 141
  secretion control 14
  stimulation test 14, 62
  thyroid profile 60
thyroid-stimulating immunoglobulins
    (TSI) 62 *see also* LATS
  Graves' disease 70, 71
thyrotrophin-releasing hormone (TRH)
    14
  TRH/LH-RH test in growth hormone
    deficiency 38–41
  and prolactin 15
  stimulation test in Graves' disease 70
  test in congenital hypopituitarism 38, 39
  triple stimulation test 19
thyroxine (T$_4$)
  -binding globulin measurement
    61
  depressed, conditions 60
  elevated, conditions 60
  normal values 142
  precocious puberty 54
  replacement 45, 65

tolbutamide stimulation
    test 135
trans-sphenoidal microadenomectomy
    99
TRH 14
tri-iodothyronine (T₃)
    conditions altered 62
    normal values 142
    reverse (rT₃) 61
    suppression test 14, 64
triple stimulation test 19, 20
    components 19
    craniopharyngioma 44, 45
    diabetes insipidus 56, 57
    extreme short stature 58, 59
    growth hormone deficiency and
        hydrocephalus 42, 43
    hypopituitarism 44, 45
    medulloblastoma radiotherapy 50, 51
    pineal germinoma 48, 49
    profile in delayed puberty 22–33
        growth hormone deficiency 36, 37
    radiation damage 46, 47
    summary chart 20
    Sustanon-primed 58
TSH *see* thyroid stimulating hormone
Turner's syndrome 18, 32, 114

ultrasound
    ovary 114
    thyroid 64

ultrasound (*cont.*)
    uterus 54
urine
    adrenocortical function 88, 89
    cAMP and phosphate 74
    glucose tests 130
    growth hormone 8
    hypocalcaemic 73
    sample collection 4, 6
    volume 4, 5

vaginoplasty 104, 108
vanillylmandelic acid 95
    normal values 143
    use 96
virus infection and growth hormone
        treatment 59
vitamin D 72–82
    intoxication 76
    metabolites in hypocalcaemia 73

water deprivation test 18
    diabetes insipidus and head injury 56,
        57
whisky stimulation test 78

Zimmermann reaction 88